STEVEN L. HIGGINS, MD, FHRS

LIVE BETTER ELECTRICALLY

Bob and Kathleen,

Thanks for you great friendship
and support for Sue and me.

Live Better Electrically,

Steve

EDITED BY: DAVID BENZ

Note to the reader: This content is not intended to be a substitute for professional medical advice, diagnosis or treatment. Your medical decisions should not be based solely on the contents of this book. Always seek the advice of your physician. The author and publisher have made reasonable efforts to determine that the recommendations meet the practice of medicine in the general medical community but do not provide any guarantees. There is no representation that drugs or device usage recommendations, including dosages, is necessarily approved by the U. S. Food and Drug Administration. Patient examples are deidentified and fictionalized to protect privacy.

Images: Images used throughout this book, unless otherwise noted, are used with permission of the author.

Library of Congress Cataloging-in-Publication Data:

Live Better Electrically: A Heart Rhythm Doc's Humorous Guide to Arrhythmias / Steven L. Higgins.

    p. cm.
    "Steven L. Higgins MD Inc."
    Includes bibliographical references and index.
    ISBN 978-0-9972360-0-2

First printing, May 2016

Contents

To Sue,

for not jumping out on Vail Pass

or since then.

Love you.

1

Introduction

The human body is an incredible machine. It is mobile, self-powered, and able to survive in all sorts of inhospitable locations. How does this machine work? Simple. Our bodies run on fuel that powers our brain and muscles. That fuel comes from what we eat and breathe, which is digested and then pumped to locations far and wide wherever it is needed. Basically, the heart is just a pump sending oxygen and other nutrients throughout the body. What's the big deal?

In 2009, while playing in a match for the soccer team KSV Roeselare, Belgian soccer player Anthony Van Loo collapsed due to ventricular fibrillation.

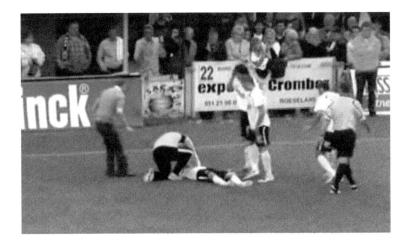

Figure 1.1: Anthony Van Loo suffers ventricular fibrillation in a 2009 soccer match. His implanted defibrillator shocked him back to life after a few seconds (Screenshot).

Van Loo described the experience afterwards:

I went after the ball. Suddenly I didn't feel very well. I reached for my head and in 3 seconds I was down. I don't remember anything after that.

After about 5 seconds, his implantable cardioverter defibrillator (ICD)—a fancy term for an implanted defibrillator—shocked his heart back into a normal rhythm. In the video, his body jolted as the defibrillator kicked in. Van Loo was essentially dead in ventricular fibrillation, only to have the defibrillator that was installed the prior year shock him back to life. Reportedly, his first words were, "Keep me in coach," or however you say that in French or Flemish.

The defibrillator worked so fast there was no damage to his brain or any other vital organs. Anthony walked off the field under his own power, and though the team doctor wouldn't let him back in the game, he joined the celebration afterwards. 50 years ago his almost instantaneous recovery couldn't ever have been thought possible. Today, we take implantable defibrillators for granted.

Our hearts beat continuously from birth to death about once a second for 2.5 billion times in a typical life. No matter whether you are thinking about your heart, distracted, asleep, in a coma or exercising, the heart keeps on beating. It happens so regularly that we often forget about this amazing organ within our bodies that keeps us alive.[1]

1.1   Awareness of heart disease

Despite incredible advances, heart disease still remains the number-one killer in the United States. In fact, it dwarfs all other causes.

More than 600,000 people die from heart disease in the United States every year (roughly one out of every four deaths).[2] It is the leading cause of death for both men and women. Heart disease is also the leading cause of death across ethnic groups.

Cancer, the most feared of illnesses, kills about half as many as heart disease. If you add strokes—a cardiac condition caused by lack of blood flow to the brain—that number is even higher.

Unfortunately, government resources go to the diseases we fear the most, breast cancer, AIDS, and so on. A sad irony is that sudden death is the biggest problem for heart disease

[1] In a repair shop, a loud-mouthed mechanic was working on a doctor's BMW. "Doc, how come you make so much money doing essentially what I do? I repair valves and electrical systems all day long, just like you." The heart doctor paused and reminded him, "Try doing it with the engine running."

[2] CDC. "Heart disease facts." 2015. http://www.cdc.gov/heartdisease/facts.htm.

research because the victim can no longer advocate for more research funding.

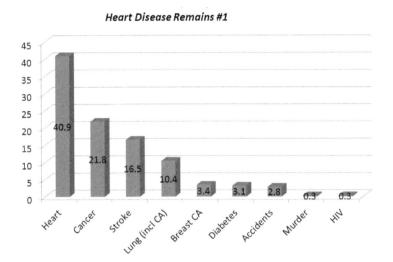

Heart Disease Remains #1

Figure 1.2: Causes of death in the United States. (Adapted from Centers for Disease Control, CDC 24/7, 2012).

In 2004, the American Heart Association (AHA) faced a challenge—half a million women a year died from heart disease, yet only 55% of women realized heart disease was their number-one threat. To help educate the public that women get heart disease, the AHA kicked off the *Go Red for Women* campaign.

Interestingly, women seem to have heart disease delayed by hormones but catch up as they age.

A study conducted after the *Go Red* public relations campaign found that women are now aware that heart disease is their leading cause of death. Still, cancer is perceived as the "greatest health risk" by a factor of three.

No doubt about it, cancer is frightening and sudden death is the way we all want to go, just not until we are 105 or so.

1.2 *Advances in heart treatments*

Despite all the gloom and doom, death from heart disease and stroke has dropped substantially.

The drop in fatalities is due to four factors:

- Awareness of the need for proper diet and exercise has improved dramatically.

- Statins (Lipitor®, Crestor®, and so on) reduce heart risk by lowering cholesterol.

- Coronary interventions from stents to emergent heart attack treatments are routinely available.

- Defibrillators save lives, whether available in an ambulance, sporting venue, or implanted internally.

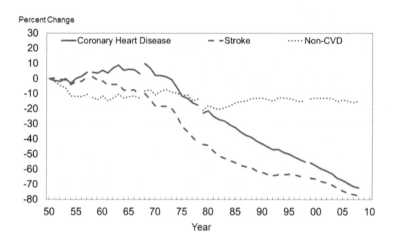

Figure 1.3: Change in mortality rates for cardiovascular (CV) and non-CV diseases in the United States, 1950-2008 (Modified from National Heart, Lung, and Blood Institute, NIH, 2010).

Despite these advances, heart disease still remains the number one killer of adult Americans.

1.3   Live better electrically

Heart disease is huge, particularly in developed countries. As a result, its management has been segmented into various specialties, including:

- General cardiologists

- Interventional cardiologists—the plumbers

- Structural heart specialists—the valve mechanics

- Heart failure specialists—the pill dispensers

- Cardiac electrophysiologists (EPs)—the electricians

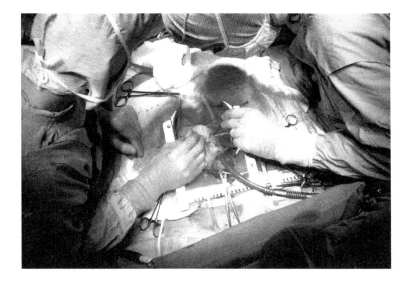

Figure 1.4: Coronary artery bypass surgery (Photo by Jerry Hecht/Wikimedia).

Cardiologists comprise the specialties outlined and all of their training starts with the nonsurgical discipline of internal medicine.

Cardiac surgeons perform major surgery on the heart. Unfortunately for them, but fortunately for the rest of us, cardiologists keep inventing less invasive ways of treating the heart without the need for an electric saw. Angioplasty and stents have often replaced the need for bypass surgery; transvenous leads passed through a vein under your collarbone have replaced the need for sewing leads and patches on the heart; transcatheter aortic valve replacement (TAVR) can avoid the need for an open procedure.[3]

I live in the world of electrical heart rhythm management. Because EP is a very specialized area, some people say that I have learned more and more about less and less such that I now know everything about nothing.

Live Better Electrically focuses on just the electrical aspects of heart care. This includes prevention, lifestyle modifications, medication options as well as the invasive treatments from implanted devices (pacemakers, defibrillators) to catheter ablation.

I put together *Live Better Electrically* to share my 35 years of experience and tell a few jokes along the way.

Live Better Electrically is organized in self-contained chapters

[3] Don't tell my heart surgeon friends, but the ultimate goal of the cardiologist is to put the open heart surgeon out of business.

that can be read sequentially or individually:[4]

- *Chapter 2:* What is an arrhythmia?

- *Chapter 3:* Symptoms—from sudden death to none at all

- *Chapter 4:* Six steps to diagnose your heart rhythm issue

- *Chapter 5:* How to document your rhythm problem

- *Chapter 6:* How to save a life with CPR

- *Chapter 7:* Arrhythmias 101: Slow and fast

- *Chapter 8:* Risk factors

- *Chapter 9:* Diet and over-the-counter drugs

- *Chapter 10:* Finding the right doctor

- *Chapter 11:* Blood thinners and prescription medications

- *Chapter 12:* Devices 1: So you need a pacemaker

- *Chapter 13:* Devices 2: So you need a defibrillator

- *Chapter 14:* Ablation

- *Chapter 15:* Safety and ablation

- *Chapter 16:* Atrial fibrillation

- *Chapter 17:* Heart failure

- *Chapter 18:* Future advances— some available today

Are you learning for yourself or a loved one and need to know about a specific issue? If so, each chapter is designed to be self-sufficient and it is all right to skip around. Do you want to increase your knowledge of arrhythmias? Then read on from the start.

[4] In 1991, Mother Teresa developed chest pain across the border at her Tijuana mission and was hospitalized at Scripps Clinic. My interventional cardiology colleague, Paul Teirstein, inserted several coronary stents to help her. After hearing of her likely future sainthood, I recently sent Paul a note, "What should I call the Jew who saved Mother Teresa, the Saint Saver?" He replied "As she reminded me at the time, 'don't forget Jesus was a Jew.' " If Mother Teresa can have such a good sense of humor about religion, I feel I can tell a few jokes about cardiology.

2

What is an arrhythmia?

As mentioned, a pump is a useful analogy for understanding the heart.

If you think of the heating system in your house as a pump, you know that it pulls in air from the outside, heats the air, and then distributes it through your house through a series of ducts. Similarly, the heart acts as a pump that circulates blood throughout your body.

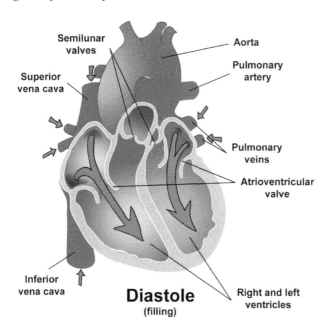

Figure 2.1: The flow of blood through a normal heart. *Diastole* is intake or filling (Modified from Mariana Ruiz Villarreal/Wikimedia).

The heart circulates blood in two cycles, a filling cycle (*diastole*—di-AS-toe-lee) and a pumping cycle (*systole*—SIS-toe-lee).

Heart valves opening and closing make the "lub dub" sound you can hear with a stethoscope.

The "lub" is made by valves closing at the beginning of systole or pumping. Systole is when the ventricles contract, or squeeze, and pump blood out of the heart. The right side of the heart sends blood to the lungs to pick up oxygen (blue in the picture shown). The left side receives oxygen-rich blood from the lungs and pumps it out to the rest of the body (red in the picture shown).

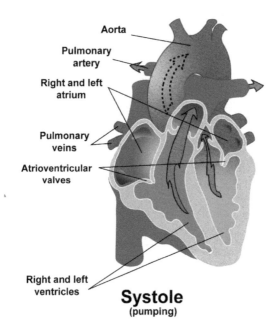

Aorta

Pulmonary artery

Right and left atrium

Pulmonary veins

Atrioventricular valves

Right and left ventricles

Systole
(pumping)

Figure 2.2: *Systole* is outflow or pumping (Modified from Mariana Ruiz Villarreal/Wikimedia).

The "dub" is made by valves closing at the beginning of diastole or filling. Diastole is when the ventricles relax and fill with blood from the atria.

Don't worry if you don't understand all of this right now. The important thing to understand is that the heart, even though it is technically a muscle, acts very similarly to how a pump works.

To keep that pump on time, the heart has an electrical system that synchronizes the intake (diastole) and the pumping (systole).

At the top of the heart is a built-in pacemaker called the sinus node, some call it the sinoatrial node or SA node. Yes, we are all born with pacemakers in our hearts. The sinus node can be influenced externally, such as with adrenaline, to drive the heart rate faster. That is why your heart beats faster when you exercise or are startled. Regardless, this sinus node has cells that have a natural capacity to beat rhythmically. This electrical signal is then transmitted throughout the upper heart chambers, called the atria. The atria are the filling chambers. I don't want to get too technical, but the right atrium is on the right and the left atrium is on the left.

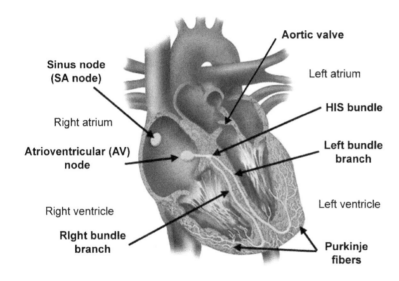

Figure 2.3: The heart's electrical system that controls the "pumping" (Modified from CEUFast.com with permission).

The heart is designed so that these electrical signals cannot get to the lower chambers, the ventricles, except through a special pathway called the atrioventricular (AV) node. Whoever designed the AV node was brilliant because problems in the atria can't easily extend into the more important lower pumping chambers.

The AV node is smart enough to know that when it's bombarded with atrial beats, such as in a common upper-chamber arrhythmia called atrial fibrillation (AF), it decreases the number that can get through. Thus, common AF cannot progress into ventricular fibrillation (VF), which causes sudden death. I told you the heart is well designed.

Below the AV node, the electrical signals travel on discrete roads, called bundle branches, so electricity actually gets to the bottom of the heart first. In the normal heart, this allows for the lower parts of the ventricles to contract first and efficiently squeeze the blood upward out the valves into the major blood vessels.

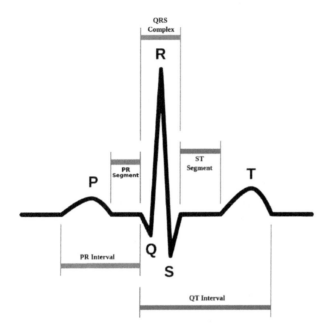

Figure 2.4: The electrical components of a normal heart beat (Image by Anthony Atkielski/Wikimedia).

The sinus node beats once a second, which causes the atria to contract, pumping blood into the ventricles. This creates a P wave on the electrocardiogram (EKG). The P wave is the atria contracting and the PR interval is the ventricles filling (diastole). The P waves that appear before each QRS are upright and the intervals between the P waves are regular.

After the ventricles have filled, the ventricular heart muscle contracts from bottom to top shooting blood out the aorta to the body. This creates the large QRS on the EKG and is when the heart is pumping. At the end of the QRS cycle, there is an interval and a T wave as the ventricles relax. Then, the cycle repeats.

This is the normal heart rhythm, also called sinus rhythm because the heartbeat's electrical impulse originates in the sinus node. It is a beautiful symphony, repeated about 100,000 times a day for each of us.

2.1   Arrhythmias

The word arrhythmia comes from the Greek a = "not" and rhythmia = "rhythm." Wait, not a heart rhythm? That doesn't seem right. More likely, it comes from Latin (or pig Latin) to mean abnormal rhythm. Seriously, there was a trend a few years ago to start calling them dysrhythmias but that never caught on. Arrhythmia just means *abnormal heart rhythm*. This diagnosis isn't necessarily serious, just abnormal—something is different than the normal EKG picture.

Although there are many heart issues, they can be simply divided into plumbing or electrical. We're going to focus on the electrical.

Looking at the depiction of the two disciplines, it doesn't take a genius to realize which job is more desirable. Heart electricians, called cardiac electrophysiologists or simply EP doctors, are the most important and handsome physicians in medicine.

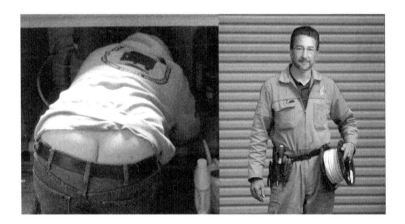

Figure 2.5: Plumbers and electricians—the two main cardiology disciplines.

Our natural sinus node pacemaker drives the normal heart's electrical system day and night, at least once a second your entire life. That is typically 2.5 billion times if you make it to age 70 or older. So, it is not surprising that occasionally there are rhythm problems.

Rhythm problems, arrhythmias, matter because the electrical system drives the heart pump. Problems with your heart rhythm can cause the pump engine to not run correctly. A major electrical problem can cause the pump motor to suddenly stop running, not a good thing if you are a heart.

2.2   *Wrap: Slow and fast arrhythmias*

One easy distinction to make when it comes to arrhythmias is between slow and fast. Heart rhythms can be slower than normal (bradycardia) or faster than normal (tachycardia).

Doctors call slow heartbeats *bradycardia* and fast heartbeats *tachycardia* to sound superior because slow and fast are too easy for you to understand.

If you promise not to tell anyone, I will share a top-secret medical lesson of the five rules we doctors are taught the first day of school:

1. Medical words must be longer than normal words.

2. Preventive medicine is bad for business.

3. If it ain't broke, don't fix it.

4. If it hurts when you do that, don't do that.

5. All you need to ever know about dermatology is, "If it's wet, dry it and if it's dry, wet it." The corollary to this is that if the dermatologist won't touch it, *don't touch it*.

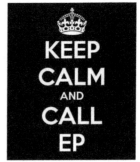

Figure 2.6: A sign designed by an EP doctor to remind his surgical colleagues that he is available to place a pacemaker when the aortic valve implant causes electrical heart block (With permission, Mintu Turakhia, MD).

Slow or fast arrhythmias often produce symptoms, such as sustained racing, fainting, or others. These symptoms are important clues as to whether an arrhythmia is serious.

In the next chapter, we'll look at these symptoms. Then we'll talk about how to diagnose your arrhythmia and get into the different types of arrhythmias in more detail. This way, you'll know when you need to see a heart electrician (EP doctor).

3
Symptoms—from sudden death to none at all

If the truth be told, doctors could medically diagnose and manage most cardiac rhythm issues over the phone if they could see the heart rhythm recording. The entire diagnosis depends on what the patient is feeling (symptoms) along with what the heart rhythm is at the time, as confirmed by an electrocardiogram (EKG).[1] However, there are many clues that can help you diagnose your own situation.

"Symptom" is the term doctors use to describe a physical or mental condition, generally considered a sign of a disease. However, symptoms vary dramatically from person to person. I have seen people wide awake claiming that nothing was wrong when their heart was in ventricular tachycardia (VT) racing at 180 beats per minute (bpm), an inch away from sudden death. Similarly, some people feel every skipped beat as if it was their last.

3.1   Syncope = fainting

The most valuable symptom in cardiac rhythm management is fainting, what doctors call *syncope*. By the way, fainting is syncope, no difference, one of the rare medical terms where the complicated medical term is shorter than what real people use (I'll bet you counted the letters, didn't you?).

Today ignoring a fainting episode is just plain wrong. Most syncope occurs because the blood flow to the brain is so low that it can't function, sort of like narcolepsy, those rare sudden sleeping attacks. This lack of blood flow can only be due to fast or slow heart rhythms or low blood pressure.

[1] I have a friend of a friend who practices radiology (reads x-rays) on the east coast but lives in Hawaii! Now, that is a commute. Actually, he works at his Hawaii condo's computer for an 8-hour shift reading x-rays during what is the middle of the night for emergency rooms in small hospitals in the Northeast. Not a bad gig, huh? In truth, most of cardiology could be done with this same telemedicine approach although wouldn't you all miss waiting in the exam room naked in a paper gown?

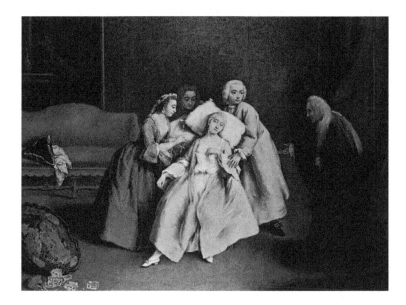

Figure 3.1: Die Ohnmacht (Fainting) by Pietro Longhi (Image courtesy Wikimedia).

In general, with fainting, gravity is our friend. With loss of control of your body, you will collapse to the floor where it might be easier for your heart to pump blood to your brain and awaken the machine. Of course, falling has its own hazards. Many a trauma patient comes in to the emergency room with all the care focused on the injury (fell off a ladder, hit his head) rather than the initial cause. If the patient is lucky, the problem will recur while on a heart monitor so treatment, such as a pacemaker, can be provided to prevent another event. In one research study, pacemakers were shown to decrease repeat fainting episodes from 60% to 5%. Of course, not everyone who faints needs a pacemaker, but certainly they need a thorough medical evaluation.

Syncope has many causes. The most common is heartbeats that are either too slow or too fast. However, other causes must be considered. It is a common public misconception that fainting is due to low blood sugar or a stroke or other neurological condition; this is exceedingly rare. Strokes might cause fainting but with other symptoms like weakness of an arm or leg. The same can be said for seizures; they might cause fainting but only with muscle jerking and prolonged confusion. People do sometimes faint from other heart problems, such as low blood pressure or a heart valve problem.[2]

Actually, we would all faint every time we stood up if it weren't for our heart and blood vessel protections. When you stand, gravity drives your blood to your feet. Instantly, a sensor in your neck, called the carotid body, realizes the pressure is low and tells the heart to beat faster at the same time that hormones are released to stimulate the heart to pump stronger and the blood vessels to constrict. In some people, that compensatory mechanism doesn't work right, so they do faint. These patients typically faint only when standing, often in a warm or crowded setting (such as at church). Treatment might be as simple as more salt and fluids or medications. That type of fainting used to be called vasovagal syncope. It can be benign (harmless) unless you happen to be the good church goer who faints and hits your head on a wooden pew. Thus, in my mind, all syncope warrants a doctor's visit for further evaluation. Fainting might be the only warning of a future risk of sudden death.

As mentioned, the most common cause of syncope is a slow or fast heartbeat. Bradycardia (slow heartbeat) occurs more commonly as we age. With other advances in medicine, the heart's own pacemaker wears out before we do. Usually, I hear, "I have always had a slow heart," as if that makes it normal. Others state they have "an athlete's heart" that causes it to go slow.[3] Seriously slow heart rhythms, often called sick sinus syndrome, progress to the point the heart is so slow you pass out. Sick sinus syndrome has a nice alliteration to it but doesn't accurately describe the reasons why many hearts go so slow they can cause fainting.

3.2   Dizziness or pre-syncope

Similar to fainting, dizziness can be insignificant or a serious warning sign sometimes referred to as "pre-syncope." It might all depend on the details. It is interesting to hear accounts of patients and witnesses when it comes to fainting. The patient often says "I didn't really pass out," while the witness says the patient collapsed to the floor and could not be aroused for a few seconds or longer. Having witnesses makes a huge difference because being unresponsive is obviously much more

[2] Low blood pressure causing fainting can be due to excessive blood pressure medication, dehydration (have you been to Arizona in July?), or other similar causes.

[3] While Olympic-level training can cause slower heart rates, the average Joe who runs 30 minutes a day for exercise is not that kind of athlete.

serious. It suggests the heart rate was so slow or fast that the blood pressure could no longer support normal brain function. It doesn't take a doctor to tell you that this experience is bad, perhaps one step from sudden death.

Thus, doctors have to take a thorough history when they hear about a dizzy spell. Was the patient just standing up from sitting or lying? Sudden position changes, such as getting up out of bed, can be associated with dizziness while our bodies adjust to the changes from gravity. Was the episode associated with prolonged standing, particularly on a hot day or when someone is dehydrated? This could be orthostatic hypotension.[4] Did you feel anything just before getting dizzy, like a rapid heart rate, chest pain, or nausea? This provides physicians more clues about the cause.

Is there evidence of trauma, such as a bruise or head trauma? Trauma evidence tells us that the faint was bad enough the patient could not protect himself, thus becoming truly unresponsive. Are there signs of a neurological cause? After the episode, continued localized weakness (one arm or leg) or slurred speech suggests a stroke. Most seizures are associated with uncontrolled shaking of extremities and/or extended confusion severe enough the patient cannot remember who or where he is. Neurological causes of dizziness or fainting are actually quite rare.[5]

Was there a warning? Diabetics can faint from a low blood sugar with too much insulin, often preceded by intense hunger, shakiness, or sweating. Low blood sugar is *not* a common explanation for dizziness or fainting in people who do not have dizziness. Just like dehydration, hypoglycemia (low blood sugar) is often used as an excuse for an event when the actual cause was a more serious arrhythmia. About half of arrhythmia patients who faint have the sensation of their heart racing just before fainting. Because the typical dizzy episode from an arrhythmia is not associated with confusion, the patient might be able to remember how he felt just before the event.

3.3   *Palpitations*

Palpitations are the most common symptom that might be related to a heart rhythm issue. "Palpitation" is the term we

[4] Orthostatic hypotension is a big medical term for when your blood pressure suddenly drops when you stand up from sitting or lying down. It is often mild, lasting no more than a few seconds. If you experience this frequently, see a doctor.

[5] Where does the stereotype of the "ditzy blond" come from? No, blonds do not have more arrhythmias. Dating back to the 1700s, the French theater first portrayed blonds as attractive but dumb, sometimes including fake fainting or swooning episodes. Scientific studies have not supported any intelligence differences between blonds and brunettes though studies have shown that blond hair color can negatively impact career advancement. A Cornell University study showed that blond waitresses received larger tips than brunettes even when controlling for other variables (age, breast size, height, and weight). Forget doing arrhythmia research, this sounds like a lot more fun. Please insert your favorite blond joke here.

doctors use when you feel either a fast or irregular heartbeat; just the sensation is what we term a palpitation. The sensation of an irregular heartbeat doesn't always mean you have one either.

Obviously, there can be many causes of palpitations. After exercising, we have all felt our hearts beating fast. Of course, that is normal because your body needs extra strong blood flow to supply your muscles with needed oxygen and nutrients. Similarly, many of us have felt a "skipped beat" commonly in the middle of the night, typically because it is so quiet then that you are not distracted from other activities. Also, when you lay on your left side, your heart is closer to your chest wall and it is easier to feel skipped beats. It is normal to have up to hundreds of these premature beats a day. Unfortunately, the more you become aware of them, the more you become aware of them.

It is important to document your heart rhythm during these symptomatic palpitations to determine whether it is a legitimate arrhythmia or a normal event. Documentation that your isolated palpitations are just normal skipped or premature beats can be immensely helpful for understanding and reassurance purposes.

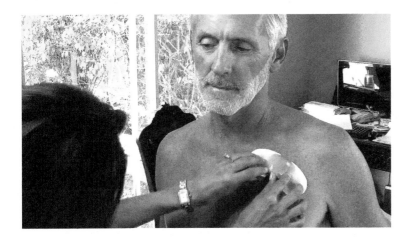

Figure 3.2: iRhythm ZIO® Patch 14-day event monitor.

More serious palpitations occur with the sensation of sustained (defined as more than 30 seconds) sudden rapid heart rates, whether regular or irregular. Regular rapid palpitations are most commonly due to a supraventricular tachycardia, often called SVT. Depending on how rapid and your general health, it can lead to syncope or other serious problems. Again, documentation is important to help with diagnosing and treating the issue. Rapid irregular palpitations are the most common symptom with atrial fibrillation (AF). If this lasts for more than just a few seconds (isolated skipped beats), it warrants a trip to the doctor for diagnosis. These days, technology can help us document our own rhythm when we have palpitations with heart rhythm monitors.

3.4 Chest pain

Chest pain is actually a relatively rare symptom of a heart *rhythm* issue, as it most commonly occurs from lack of blood flow to the heart. Chest pain unrelated to dizziness is often another issue, typically a reason to see the heart plumber and get your pipes fixed. Think about it, if your heart is not beating effectively from an arrhythmia, you might not get enough blood flow to your brain and thus the sensation of dizziness, or to your heart, and the sensation of chest pain. Some people even get belly pain from lack of blood flow from an arrhythmia.

In medical school, physicians are taught that heart pain can cause pain anywhere from the belly button to the chin. Do you know why? The inner organs, unlike our skin, have no sensory nerves. So, when something goes wrong, like lack of oxygen to the heart, the pain is "referred" to nerves elsewhere. Most people commonly get left arm pain referred from their heart.

3.5 Normal heart rate range

What is a normal heart rate? At rest, adults typically have a heart rate between 60 and 80 bpm. When asleep, it might slow even further, commonly into the 50s and rarely 40s. Of course, certain normal conditions will cause faster heart rates, such as activity, fever, anxiety, first love, and so on. Other non-cardiac medical issues can make a normal heart go faster at rest, such as an overactive thyroid or tumors or many other causes.

What is the deal with love and the heart anyway? To be honest, there is no clear explanation of why the heart is associated with love. It is likely part ancient history, part superstition, and

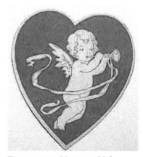

Figure 3.3: Vintage Valentine's Day card (Image by Dave/Flickr).

part a modern gift card sales opportunity. Of course, anything that can stimulate the body to release adrenaline will increase the heart rate and, certainly, a first date can provoke anxiety and adrenaline release. Physiologists tell us that a natural part of courting includes adrenaline release to bring blood to the skin and lips.

Similarly, why a Valentine's Day image of the heart? Most people are aware the human heart is actually more like a large fist in shape. Some have speculated the heart shape is related to a woman's cleavage, which is a lot more romantic than a fist. While we are on this topic, why is it romantic to have an arrow in your heart depicting love? Your guess is as good as mine.

Some believe the heart and love connection arose from an early belief that the heart was the center of emotion and think-ing (those ancient prophets were so naive because scientists today have proven that *thinking* has nothing to do with love). Medieval art as far back as the 13th century depicted suitors giving their heart (yes, an actual heart) to a lady. The ancient Greek physician Galen claimed the liver was the seat of the soul and emotions. Hallmark would never sell a card with a picture of a liver.

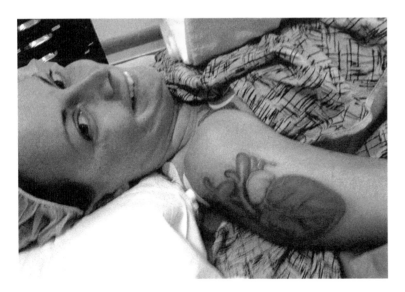

Figure 3.4: Patient with a heart tattoo on the day of her ablation (Photo with patient permission).

Several years ago, I did a catheter ablation procedure on a young woman with dangerous heart racing. This woman had a tattoo of an anatomically correct heart placed on her shoulder, complete with arteries, valves, and so on. The tattoo artist added an arrow that actually pierced the tattooed heart in the very spot the arrhythmia originated. As part of the ablation, we created a 3-D color anatomic model of the inside of the heart. I sent the 3-D image along with a photo of the heart tattoo to the prestigious New England Journal of Medicine for their "Images in Medicine" section. Those boring editors rejected it; no sense of humor!

What is a normal heart rate with activity? As long as you don't have medication or other reasons for a slower-than-normal heart, the age-old formula holds amazingly true:

Maximum heart rate = 220 − your age.

The maximum is what you would achieve with a sudden burst of activity, such as running a 50-yard dash, which can be sustained only for seconds. Assuming you aren't doing that type of activity, a more normal maximum heart rate is 70 to 80% of that number. In fact, that is the way physicians and exercise physiologists recommend training heart rate goals with exercise. For example, a 50 year old can achieve a heart rate of 170 with a sprint—220 minus 50 is 170. However, with more prolonged activity, the goal should be 70 to 80% of that or, 120 to 135 bpm. It is generally taught that if you exceed the 80% number, you actually do not achieve as much cardiac or weight loss benefit because your body becomes anaerobic.[6] Anaerobic exercise might have some value for strength training but the "burn" you feel from this type of exercise is your muscles telling you that lactic acid is building up from lack of adequate oxygen. The old adage "no pain, no gain" refers to building big muscles, not preventing heart disease.

[6] Anaerobic means "without oxygen" burning short-term energy reserves only.

The older we get, the slower our hearts beat normally. As a result, there is less safety margin from normal to dangerously slow rates. Syncope from bradycardia is common in elderly people and can be disastrous.

Physicians often see a functioning elderly person faint and sustain a hip fracture or head trauma. In advanced years, this might be the end of our ability to function independently (a nice way of saying you might need to move to an assisted living home). Thus, it is critical, particularly in the elderly, to diagnose the slow heart rhythm before the injury occurs. Unfortunately, there are no safe medications to speed up the heart, so the standard treatment is an implanted pacemaker. These days, pacemakers come in several varieties, even hidden without a surgical scar or leads. A pacemaker just reminds a slow heart to beat faster and typically cures fainting.

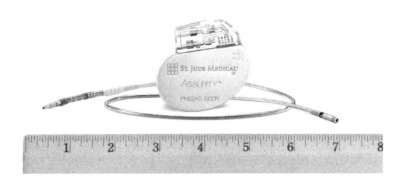

Figure 3.5: An artificial pacemaker with electrode (With permission, St. Jude Medical).

Another common cause for syncope is a fast heartbeat. Sort of like the tortoise and the hare story; when your heart races fast, it isn't as efficient as when it pumps in a normal range. At 60 bpm your heart has about a second to fill with blood, which is then pumped effectively throughout your body. At 180 bpm, that would be one-third of a second, not long enough for enough blood to flow into the pump, thus resulting in ineffective output, low blood pressure, and fainting. This type of heart racing can begin in the upper chambers, called supraventricular tachycardia (SVT), or lower chambers, ventricular tachycardia (VT). Atrial fibrillation (AF) is the most common cause of fast heart beats, an upper chamber arrhythmia, which is irregular (jumps all over when you check your pulse). Any of these causes is potentially serious and warrants a trip to a heart specialist.

3.6   Sudden death

Now, that term gets your attention, doesn't it? My professional life is the treatment of sudden death, so I take it for granted. Sudden death is the term physicians use for sudden cardiac collapse.[7] It is differentiated from syncope (fainting) because you don't wake up unless there is prompt treatment, such as a paramedic's defibrillator shock.

Sudden death is *not* a heart attack. It drives us EP doctors crazy to read in the paper about the famous person who died suddenly of a "heart attack." These reports include James Gandolfini, Justice Antonin Scalia, and many others. Usually, that is incorrect.

Only about one in three sudden death events is actually due to a heart attack, the term for a sudden blockage of an artery providing oxygen to part of the heart. The other two-thirds of sudden deaths are from an arrhythmia unrelated to an immediate heart attack. Abrupt heart artery blockage, causing a heart attack, typically causes chest pain first. Only if the area of the heart that is stressed from the blockage also has an arrhythmia does it cause sudden death. These days, most large hospitals have 24-hour teams available to promptly open up the heart artery blockage and prevent more heart muscle from dying.[8]

Don't get me wrong, heart attacks are bad, just not as bad as sudden death. Heart attacks, if untreated, cause a portion of the heart muscle to die, making it permanently weaker. This event can cause heart failure symptoms, such as shortness of breath and fatigue. Scars associated with this dead heart muscle are the most common cause of sudden death (typically years after the heart attack). Two in three sudden deaths are due to such scars in the heart or other heart muscle problems, which can be associated with development of a sudden life-threatening lower chamber (ventricular) arrhythmia.

How strange is this? Just now, I had to stop writing to take a call from the wife of a patient who died recently. Twenty five years ago, he received his first implanted defibrillator by me, and required five revisions or replacements over the years. While these defibrillators prevented sudden death, this man continued on to develop heart failure with severe fatigue and shortness of breath. Fortunately, medical technology had again advanced so he received something we will discuss later called cardiac resynchronization therapy (CRT). Unfortunately, in recent years, age and his weakened heart limited his ability to get around. He was even offered an artificial heart but refused.

[7] Sudden Death is also the name of my Fantasy Football team.

[8] The goal is to treat these heart attacks, called STEMIs (ST segment elevation myocardial infarction), promptly with a "door to balloon" time of less than 90 minutes. As the interventional cardiologists love to say, "Time is muscle." Thus if you are having chest pain, get to the hospital or emergency clinic as quickly as possible.

Finally, at age 87, he had an exacerbation of his heart failure and died peacefully in the hospital. While this was officially a sudden death, it took more than 25 years to play itself out.[9]

Although it might be sudden, sudden death is not the term used for suddenly dying from other non-cardiac causes, such as getting hit by a bus or suddenly rupturing an aneurysm. Physicians should really use the term sudden *cardiac* death for what we are discussing. Regardless, we are referring to the sudden development of a life-threatening arrhythmia. Most commonly, this rhythm problem is ventricular fibrillation (VF), a totally disorganizing quivering of the heart which stops the heart from pumping blood with its life saving oxygen to the entire body.

[9] Amazingly, this Hispanic man was named Jesus. On the call, Jesus's wife was very appreciative of how his life had been extended, recalling that I had quoted a 50% chance of dying within 5 years more than two decades ago. I don't mind being wrong like *that*.

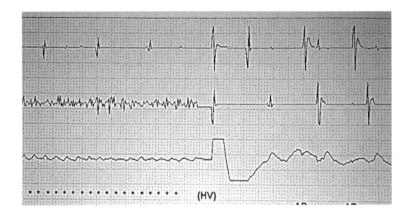

Figure 3.6: The development of VF terminated by an implanted defibrillator high voltage shock within 8 seconds.

If you look at the second line of the EKG shown, it doesn't take a cardiologist to tell you that something is wrong. The heart is in a life-threatening heart rhythm, ventricular fibrillation, with totally disorganized electrical activity. This means it is just quivering, unable to pump blood anywhere; death would happen in another minute or 2. Fortunately, this patient was saved by an implanted defibrillator within a matter of seconds. Other than a surprise shock, the patient is fine—a great example of "living better electrically."

Recently, I took care of a lucky man who was working at a coffee cart outside a local community hospital. He collapsed in front of doctors and nurses waiting for their triple venti soy, no foam, extra-hot lattes. Cardiopulmonary resuscitation (CPR) was initiated, a defibrillator arrived, and he was shocked back into regular rhythm. In the emergency room, he was stabilized.[10] EKGs and blood tests could not exclude a heart attack, so the heart attack or STEMI protocol was initiated.

The barista was promptly transported to Scripps Hospital where at emergent cardiac catheterization his heart arteries were found to be diseased, so they were propped open with stents. However, the arteries were not completely blocked as is seen in a true STEMI (heart attack) but severely narrowed. In medicine we refer to this as the surgeon's mantra "a chance to cut is a chance to cure." Of course, this patient likely will do better with stents keeping him from future heart attacks, but this event was not why he collapsed making the latte. An echocardiogram (heart ultrasound) study revealed that his heart was weak and scarred from previous heart attacks because he had what we call an ischemic cardiomyopathy.[11] Research has shown that anyone with a weak heart is at increased risk of sudden death. Before hospital discharge, the barista received an implantable defibrillator and continues to do well.

[10] Some hospitals have tried to change the name of the emergency room to the emergency department because it has many more than one room but the name change never seems to catch on.

[11] *Ischemic cardiomyopathy* is a fancy medical term for a weak heart from prior heart attacks.

3.7   No symptoms

As Donald Rumsfeld explained, the unknown unknowns can be worse than the known unknowns. This saying could be applied to cardiac symptoms too. About 50% of serious arrhythmia patients show no symptoms. Sometimes patients simply are unwilling to admit to any symptoms. More commonly, however, people really don't feel the heart rhythm problem. Many times, this is a good thing because you are able to function without the distraction of constant concern about your heart.

Today, we commonly do continuous heart monitors. It never ceases to amaze me how many serious rapid or slow arrhythmias occur in people who are completely unaware. Of course, just because you don't feel it doesn't make a heart rate of 200 bpm any less dangerous. For example, your very first symptom could be a fatal car crash. In fact, no one knows how many unexplained car accidents are due to the driver having a sudden arrhythmia, "He just swerved into my lane." Even the more benign upper chamber arrhythmias, such as SVT and AF, can result in sudden death if you extend that term to include fainting and the resultant trauma.

3.8   Red herring symptoms

That term is pretty silly, isn't it? Supposedly it originally had something to do with stinky fish distracting a hunting dog from the trail. Regardless, we now use red herring to mean misleading findings, similar to the expression "true-true, unrelated." The physician's job, and yours too, is to figure out if the symptoms you experience are related to something serious or just a random sensation to be ignored.

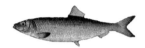

Figure 3.7: An actual red herring (Screenshot).

Red herring symptoms are those that sound like they could be serious but aren't. Again, modern technology has helped tremendously with this issue. Event and Holter monitors allow us to record heart rhythms for extended times outside of the medical office. When associated with an ability to document the heart rhythm at the exact instance of a symptom (an event button is pressed while the EKG is being recorded), it can be quite revealing. The famous 80:20 rule applies here. When people feel palpitations, about 80% of the time, they have a real arrhythmia. Of course, that arrhythmia might be benign, such as rare isolated premature beats, but they are nevertheless feeling something real. However, 20% of the time, people will state, "I feel it now," and their heart rhythm is entirely normal. Not all of these people need to lie down on a couch with a good psychiatrist.[12] Actually, the ability to demonstrate to such a person that his symptoms are red herrings, totally misleading, and unrelated to any serious heart issue, can itself be healing. Reassurance from a learned person in a white coat is a time-honored medical treatment.

Perfectly normal people can believe that they are having a serious heart rhythm issue when they are not. Making it even more complicated, this can occur in people who also have had serious arrhythmias at other times. This experience causes them to focus on their heart rhythm. Sometimes, these imaginary symptoms can be as disabling as real problems. Treating this issue can be challenging because patients don't come to the doctor to be told it's not real. However, the mind that is powerful enough to imagine events can treat them too.

Using biofeedback often works in managing symptoms unrelated to serious heart issues. Biofeedback is the process of gaining greater awareness of your own body. It is helpful to

[12] A guy gets a flat tire in front of a mental hospital. One patient watches him as he jacks up the car and takes the tire off. He installs the spare tire but as he is reaching for the lug nuts, they fall into a nearby storm drain.

The patient says, "Psst, mister. Need some help?" The guy who is now stranded says, "How could you possibly help me with this problem?" The patient replies, "Take a bolt from each of your other three wheels, reattach the spare tire and you should be able to safely drive to a repair shop."

The motorist replies, "What a great idea!" He then adds, "Tell me, how is such a brilliant mind locked up in a mental hospital?" The patient replies, "Well, I might be crazy but I'm not stupid."

have patients verbalize, actually saying out loud, "This is normal, no cause for concern." This technique works for many people. After using these biofeedback techniques for a few days or weeks, many patients will no longer *feel* their palpitations; problem solved.

3.9   Wrap

In medicine, some symptoms are clearly understood. If your knee hurts, you see a doctor to get it treated. In cardiology, symptoms are more variable. Some are dramatic like sudden death.[13] Fortunately, today, many sudden deaths don't really end up with death thanks to CPR and other modern advances.

Other less dramatic symptoms might also be important warnings of heart rhythm issues. Fainting, which doctors call syncope, is often a warning of a life-threatening arrhythmia. Even though you might wake up from the faint feeling fine, this generally warrants a thorough and prompt evaluation. Near-syncope is the term used for symptoms varying from dizziness to almost fainting. This too warrants medical evaluation with the significance often dependent on documentation of the heart rhythm at the time of the event.[14]

The most common symptom of an arrhythmia is palpitations, the term used for that sensation of your heart skipping a beat or racing. However, just because you feel something unusual doesn't mean that you have a serious arrhythmia, or in fact, any arrhythmia at all. Finally, some patients might have serious heart rhythm issues without any symptoms. Just because you can't feel it, doesn't mean it's always safe.

As my sister-in-law tells her children, "Sorry, kids, but today is not get-what-you-want day, it is get-what-you-get day." The same goes for heart symptoms. Doctors have to start with what the patient feels and can describe to us. Some patients can feel symptoms that are very helpful in sorting out the cause, such as "Doc, I bent over and suddenly my heart raced rapidly and regularly at a rate of 180. It stopped suddenly about 5 minutes later." Others can have the same exact arrhythmia and just not feel it. Fortunately, there are other ways to determine if there is a heart rhythm issue.

[13] *Sudden death* is the term used for the sudden collapse observed from a life-threatening arrhythmia like ventricular fibrillation.

[14] A family practitioner, an internist, a surgeon, and a pathologist are duck hunting. The family practitioner sees a duck, aims his gun, and says, "That looks like a duck, it quacks like a duck, it must be a duck." The internist looks and says "Yeah, that could be a duck. Rule out penguin, rule out flamingo, rule out ostrich. Duck versus goose seems most likely." The surgeon, firing from the hip, unloads his gun, spraying bullets all over the field. He reloads, and keeps shooting until he's empty. He then turns to the pathologist and says, "Go see if that was a duck."

4
Six steps to diagnose your heart rhythm issue

Remember the IBM computer that won *Jeopardy*? Its name was
Watson, named after the first IBM CEO. It cost more than $1
billion to develop the artificial intelligence needed to beat Ken
Jennings and receive the $1 million Jeopardy prize (subse-
quently donated to charity).

Flush with that victory, Watson decided he could win just as
easily in medicine, teaching himself to be a doctor and guide
treatment. To break it gently to those of us with an MD degree,
he is called a "clinical decision support solution." IBM and
Watson learned that medicine is not all science and that the art
of medicine, as well as cynicism, are much harder to learn.

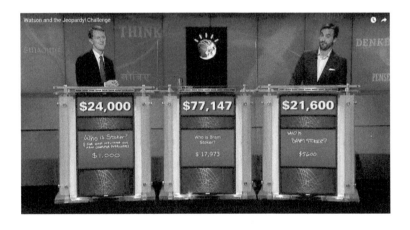

Figure 4.1: Ken Jennings
and Brad Rutter, two of the
greatest *Jeopardy* champs
ever, compete against IBM's
Watson computer in 2011
(Screenshot).

If Watson can't figure out medicine, how can I create an
algorithm that will help you?[1]

Medical diagnosis tends to follow the 80/20—80% of diag-

[1] Have you called a doctor's
office lately? You get a
machine (not nearly as
bright as Watson) and it
says, "If you are having a
life-threatening emergency,
call 911." As if you needed
to call the doctor's office to
learn that.

noses come from 20% of cases. In other words, a few situations account for most people's issues. MDs like me develop steps to identify these most common cases and these steps might give you some idea about your situation.

Before explaining the steps, here's a disclaimer: They don't pretend to cure or solve heart rhythm problems. This is just a tool to try to identify, not to cure or solve, heart rhythm problems. If you think you may have an arrhythmia, please see a doctor.

4.1   *Do you have symptoms, such as fainting?*

If your symptoms are severe, such as syncope especially with trauma or persistent chest pain, go to an emergency room (ER) or doctor for immediate evaluation. By the way, urgent care centers don't do well with most arrhythmias and will just send you on to the ER so skip that step. If your symptoms are less severe, then move to step 2. By the way, symptoms can be anything including palpitations, dizziness, feeling a funny pulse rate, shortness of breath, non-exertional chest pain, and so on.

4.2   *Do your symptoms happen doing one thing?*

Then, don't do that! That will be $50 for the advice; you're welcome.[2]

Seriously, if your symptoms happen with exercise (or always right after), then a treadmill study where your rhythm is recorded with exercise is helpful. Similarly, if you find a correlation with certain positions or activity (like bending over), mention that to your physician and intentionally try to bring on the problem when you have a heart monitor recording your rhythm. Knowledge is power.

4.3   *How regularly do your symptoms occur?*

If they are present continuously, document your problem with an EKG and physical exam at the same time. Make an appointment to see your primary care doctor. If symptoms are infrequent, then the frequency determines the next step.

[2] "Doctor, every time I have a cup of coffee, I get this stabbing pain in my right eye." The doctor replies, "Take the spoon out!"

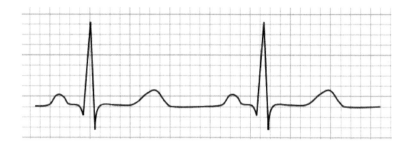

Figure 4.2: Picture of a normal EKG rhythm that you have probably seen from medical shows (Image by Madhero88/Wikimedia).

I must say that coming to a doctor's office seems to make everyone's blood pressure rise (a phenomenon called white-coat syndrome) but also everyone's arrhythmia disappear, especially when the EKG machine is on. This is similar to that crazy noise from your car that disappears when you take it into the shop.

Fortunately, technology has provided some options for remotely documenting symptoms. One example is the AliveCor Kardia™ monitor. Smaller than a credit card, the Kardia monitor allows you to capture a medical-grade EKG in just 30-seconds. This monitor then connects to an app on your smartphone that allows you to see the recordings. An Apple Watch version of Kardia called Kardia™ Band is also scheduled for release soon.

If you think your pulse is fast or slow when it shouldn't be, a recorded diary of your symptoms and your heart rate can significantly help doctors if your symptoms are sporadic. Newer technology, like the Fitbit®, can also provide valuable documentation of your heart rates, but a real EKG from something like a Kardia™ monitor is better.

If your symptoms are infrequent, your doctor might prescribe a long-term event monitor. Monitors vary from the 2-week big BAND-AID-like device called a ZIO® Patch to a continuously recording monitor, called an event monitor or mobile cardiac outpatient telemetry (MCOT).

Because it takes a few weeks to see most doctors for a routine new patient visit, it might save time to get a ZIO® Patch or a 24-hour Holter monitor before the visit so there is data to review. Be proactive when making your appointment and ask about options.

The next chapter discusses these options and devices for documenting your rhythm issue in more depth.

4.4 Did previous attempts fail to document the problem?

In general, when attempts to document the problem aren't successful, the issue falls into one of two categories: a) psychiatric and b) difficult to detect and document.

4.4.1 Psychiatric or neurological causes, including anxiety

If your symptoms occurred and your rhythm was documented to be normal, then you must accept that what you are feeling is not a heart rhythm problem. The great majority of such cases are anxiety related, though it can be based in a real sensed arrhythmia, albeit minor, such as an isolated early beat.

Unfortunately, psychiatric issues, including anxiety, are often what we call a "diagnosis of exclusion," meaning you have to rule out other medical problems first. So, if for example, your rhythm is fine but you feel severe dizziness, near or true syncope, then it is important to evaluate your blood pressure while you are having your symptoms, either with a cuff you purchase from the drug store or a prescribed automated system your doctor can provide. We need to exclude that the symptoms are not from low blood pressure without an arrhythmia. Checking your blood pressure after you have fainted is rarely of help because it usually normalizes quickly after the faint. Same for an EKG. It is much better to have a recording of your heart when the problem occurs, not after.

If the severe symptoms persist and are not anxiety or panic attacks, then a neurological workup might be appropriate (EEG, head CT scan or MRI, or neurologist exam). Nevertheless, the vast majority of patients with normal rhythms and symptoms are just anxious. In that setting, medications are rarely needed. The first step is to try the mind-over-matter approach of *biofeedback*. When you are having your concerns, tell yourself, preferably out loud, "This is normal, nothing is wrong." As weird as it sounds, your body often responds to this biofeedback and the sensation and anxiety will go away with time.[3]

[3] Biofeedback sounds so much better than "talking to yourself."

4.4.2   Difficult to detect and document

So what do you do if you are having severe symptoms and the monitors have not been able to document an event? For example, you might have worn a ZIO® Patch for 2 weeks, had no issues and the day after, had another possible rhythm related symptom. There is another technology solution available though you might not like it.

The Medtronic Reveal LINQ™ is an implantable loop recorder. It is often called "injectable" because it is so small, the delivery system is a large syringe. The LINQ™ is just 4 x 7 x 45 mm in size (about 1/4 inch wide by 1 3/4 inches long) that is implanted, "injected" in the skin.

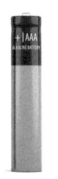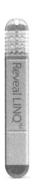

Figure 4.3: The Medtronic Reveal LINQ™ implantable loop recorder (With permission, Medtronic).

LINQ™ insertion leaves a minor scar (less than 1/2 inch) but is otherwise generally not noticeable.[4] It continuously records your heart rhythm for up to 3 years, so if you only faint once a year, this could finally pinpoint the reason. However, the LINQ™ is just a diagnostic tool and doesn't pace or treat the problem in any way. Nevertheless, figuring out the problem is critical before you can get it properly treated.

4.5   What happens if you have no symptoms?

Having your heart rhythm evaluated anyway is often a good idea. Up to 50% of patients with serious arrhythmias are completely unaware. While it might seem nice to have a warning system to know when a problem is there (for example, so that you could pull over when driving), this can sometimes be a

[4] "Not noticeable" depends on your frame of reference. Mikhail Gorbachev, the Russian leader in Ronald Reagan's time, had a giant red birthmark on his forehead that looked like a sick seagull pelted him. His subjects would say, "Gorby, don't worry, it's hardly noticeable." Same goes for that LINQ™ scar. Some are not happy about the scar; others couldn't care less.

curse. People who feel their rhythm problems can become anxious about the issue, often to their detriment. So, never fail, technology to the rescue again. Obviously a symptom-guided recording, such as an AliveCor Kardia™ smartphone monitor won't help if you don't have symptoms to know when the rhythm is abnormal. In that setting, a continuous monitor is necessary, such as a 24-hour Holter monitor or a 2-week ZIO® Patch.

4.6   Wrap: You have a diagnosis. What's next?

If you have symptoms but infrequent isolated beats (less than 5,000 a day), the best treatment is often none.

If your heart rate is slow or fast, read *Chapter 7: Arrhythmias 101: Slow and fast* and *Chapter 12: Devices 1: So you need a pacemaker* whether you need a pacemaker or not.

If you have AF, you are doomed (just kidding). AF is discussed in its own chapter and the various treatments are included in several others—medications to devices to ablation.

You will also want to talk with your doctor about your issue. This algorithm just provides some general guidelines.[5]

[5] "I saw a patient last month who fell into an upholstery machine. Fortunately, he's now fully recovered."

5
How to document your rhythm problem

If I was writing this chapter 120 years ago, I'd already be done. However, in 1903, a Dutch doctor, Willem Einthoven, invented the electrocardiogram (EKG). Of course, he foolishly called it an EKG, not ECG, so it took more than 20 years to get his Nobel Prize awarded just before his death.

Dr. Einthoven, the inventor of the EKG, recognized that the heart runs from electrical activity and that it is possible to measure that electricity with electrodes on the skin.[1]

5.1   The EKG

Documentation is key in the electrophysiology (EP) world. We need to know what your heart rhythm is doing when you complain of symptoms like fainting, benign "flip-flops," or something else. Today, with many modern advances, patients can take charge of their own health care and document their heart rhythm before they can even get in to see their doctor. Let's look at some of these ways to record what is going on with your heart.

First of all, an EKG is an ECG, no difference. Einthoven called it an electrokardiogram (EKG), in English electrocardiogram (ECG), but to this day we still often abbreviate it as EKG rather than ECG. An EKG refers to any heart rhythm recording.

Today, when using the term EKG, doctors often mean a *12-lead EKG*, the most common form of EKG where the technician hooks up stickies to your extremities and chest and records your heart rhythm from 12 different views. The first six leads are derived from different views using the extremity electrodes,

[1] Remember rule number five from the first day of med school: "All you need to ever know about dermatology is that if it is wet, dry it, and dry, wet it." Fortunately, Dr. Einthoven was there for his first day of med school and was awake. Thus, early EKGs used suction cups with liquid or gel to improve contact with the dry skin that doesn't conduct electricity well on its own.

which incidentally work just as well if you record from your hand, wrist, or shoulder. For example, Lead I just measures the electricity available from the left arm compared to the right arm electrode only.

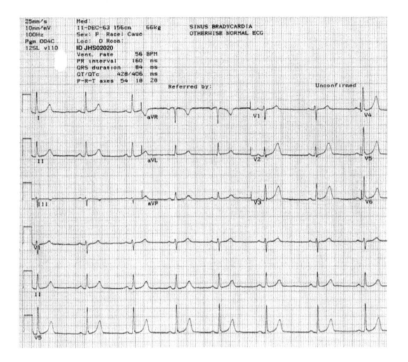

Figure 5.1: A 12-lead EKG (This one includes 12 leads on the first three lines as well as the two bottom lines, which are rhythm strip type recordings).

The last six of the 12 EKG leads are from the electrodes on specific locations on the chest wall and are compared to the limb leads electrically. We also use the term "rhythm strip" to distinguish a single channel recording from a 12-lead EKG.[2]

If you are mostly concerned with the rhythm, why do you need a big machine on a cart and all those wires? You don't. With today's technology there are an incredible number of ways to record an EKG rhythm strip.

[2] A rhythm strip is a single channel view of the heart's electrical activity. Most times, we are only concerned with the rhythm—is it regular or irregular, fast or slow?—so any window is usually adequate.

5.2   24-hour Holter monitor

Invented more than 60 years ago, the 24-hour Holter monitor became a huge advance when biophysicist and inventor, Norman "Jeff" Holter (I'd go by Jeff too) revolutionized cardiology with a continuous recording of EKG data from a patient while mobile. With the advent of transistors, the product was small enough to fit in a coat pocket, patented in 1965 and sold to Del Mar Avionics.

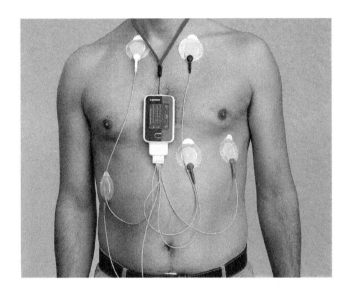

Figure 5.2: A typical 24-hour Holter monitor hookup, which also makes the other kind of hookup unlikely (Photo by Miss-curry/Wikimedia).

In an incredible coincidence, Jeff is now retired and lounging on a beach in Del Mar, California. The 24-hour Holter monitor became ubiquitous in the cardiologist's office, prescribed to patients to wear at home for 24 hours, helping to uncover intermittent arrhythmias.

Several years ago, I published a medical article asking, "Is the Holter monitor obsolete?" To save you the trouble, the answer is *yes*.[3] It only records for 24 hours at a time. This limits documentation to rhythm problems that crop up every day. It is also cumbersome. No one wants to go to work with patches on their chest, wires coming out, and a giant box on your hip. "So, Joe, I guess cruising for chicks is out tonight, eh?" The Holter lives on today only because the billing codes are established. With so many better options available, Jeff's old Holter monitor should be obsolete.

[3] Higgins, Steven L. "A novel patch for heart rhythm monitoring. Is the Holter monitor obsolete?" *Future Cardiology*, 9(3):325-333, February 2013.

5.3   ZIO® Patch

In 2006, a young, nerdy EP doc, like me but younger and more handsome, with the help of the Stanford University Biodesign program, created what entrepreneurs call a "disruptive techno-logical advance." That nerd is a friend of mine, Uday Kumar, MD, who developed and commercialized the ZIO® Patch, by iRhythm Technologies.

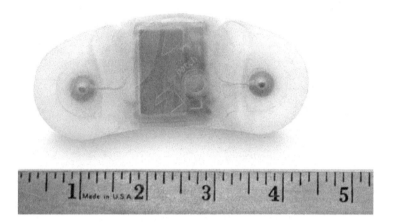

Figure 5.3: A wireless ZIO® Patch 14-day event monitor (With permission, iRhythm Technologies).

The ZIO® Patch has been described as a "Big BAND-AID" easily stuck on the upper chest where it records the same heart rhythm as a 24-hour Holter monitor, without any visible wires, and in addition does it continuously for up to 14 days! This ZIO® Patch has become a huge advance in cardiology, copied by competitors and welcomed by patients because it can be hidden under clothes, worn in the shower, and mailed back for interpretation, avoiding another trip to the doctor's office.

5.4 AliveCor Kardia™

Another incredibly simple and easy-to-use advance is the AliveCor Kardia™ heart monitor. To get this, you don't need a prescription or doctor visit. In fact, you can even buy them on Amazon for about $75. AliveCor Kardia™ supplies a case for your smartphone and you place a couple of fingers on each metal electrode and can see your own EKG live.

To make more than $75, AliveCor has developed an optional service to read your EKG too, a pretty clever idea. Unlike a ZIO® Patch, which is continuously recording, you have to acti-vate the AliveCor Kardia™ to record your EKG. However, you can save your exact rhythm at the time of your symptoms. So,

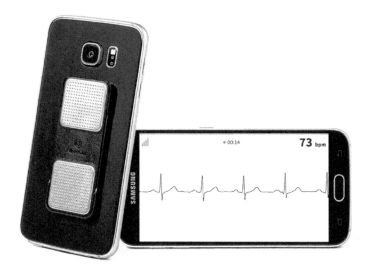

Figure 5.4: An AliveCor smartphone case and display of an EKG (With permission, AliveCor, Inc).

if you feel your heart racing, this is a great tool to document the rate and show your doctor the EKG to prove that you really aren't nuts. By the way, there are several good competitors to AliveCor out there, Cardiac Designs™ ECG Check, the Heart Check™ PEN and others. However, your typical phone app is not as good as these actual EKG recording systems.

Not long after this tool first became available, they were kind enough to send me one (saving a whopping $75 because I am a "key opinion leader"). Not long after, I was at a local restaurant for a meeting having some delicious wine with friends when someone shouted, "Steve, come check out Ruth, she doesn't look so hot." Boy, were they right. Still upright in her chair, Ruth was essentially dead. She was pulseless, not breathing, and that pale gray color you don't want to get unless you're dressing up as a zombie for Halloween.

I quickly moved her to the floor (unfortunately banging her head on the thin carpet) and started CPR (remember "Stayin' Alive, Stayin' Alive, Ah, ah, ah, ah ..."). Amazingly, Ruth began to wake up! I pulled out my phone and recorded an EKG with my Kardia™ app showing a heart rate of 35 (better than the rate of zero I had noted a minute prior when feeling for a pulse). Fortunately, I documented this as her heart rate promptly normalized. By the way, the same electrodes on the Kardia™ case work just fine if you place it directly on the chest. After awakening, Ruth's first words were, "No big deal. I've had this for a long time. I always wake up."[4] Ruth also wasn't happy with my insistence that she go in an ambulance to the hospital, and even less happy to get a pacemaker implanted the next day.

I think she remains unhappy with me even though those nasty fainting spells have stopped.

[4] You always wake up until you don't. Don't be like Ruth. See a doctor if you faint.

5.5   Heart rate monitors

There must be a million heart rate monitors available now. They come in standalone versions, like Fitbit®, Polar monitors, and New Balance, most designed for jocks. They also come as free or paid apps to smartphones, smartwatches, and so on. On the watches, they use a sensor that touches the skin of one arm. On the phones, some use the camera flash as a light to look for pulsations in your fingertip. I know you don't want to hear about them all.

Most of the time, these devices are fine for getting an approximate number of your heart rate. However, they often make mistakes, particularly if your rhythm is not regular. While these monitors are great if you just want to know how fast your pulse is (and don't have a watch with a second hand), they are no substitutes for EKGs, particularly when you can store the recording for later review.

5.6   Event recorders and mobile cardiac outpatient telemetry (MCOT)

Again, not to belabor the point, but there are also other medical options to the 24-hour Holter monitor that can provide recordings of your heart rhythm. These include something called an event recorder, which can continuously track your rhythm, most commonly with wires attached for an extended time. When you have a symptom, even something as serious as syncope, you can press a button and it will store the loop of EKGs for the prior minute or two.

An MCOT is a device that records your rhythm continuously and, through the miracles of today's cell phone technology, sends it to a monitoring center in real time. At the center, some incredibly bored guy is watching your monitor in case you have a dangerous arrhythmia. In some ways, the real-time nature is better than a ZIO® Patch, which you must remove and mail in before anyone sees your heart rhythm. However, MCOTs are more expensive, have wires (at least most do today), and require an accurate monitoring center. In addition, MCOTs can't fix issues. They just diagnose the rhythm problem. "Yup, he went into VF and died. At least we got his insurance info up front." Sometimes this type of telemetry is better reserved for in the hospital.

5.7   Implantable loop recorder

The implantable loop recorder is a surgical alternative to diagnose rhythm problems when it is *really* a mystery. The technology for this advance is pretty cool; essentially it is so small it is injectable, though the implanted device does leave a scar. Also note that this device only establishes what the rhythm issue is without doing anything to correct it.

5.8   Wrap

If you or a loved one (or even just a liked one) have a heart rhythm issue, the key is documentation. Of course, you shouldn't delay seeing a physician but you can be proactive by attempting to document your heart rhythm at the time you have your symptoms. I love it when a patient brings to me his own recording of his heart rhythm. It makes it that much easier to proceed to treatment.

Here are some general guidelines to help with documenting your heart rhythm:

- If you just want to know your heart rate, particularly when exercising, get a heart rate monitor.

- If you have an intermittent rhythm issue, see a physician to get a regular EKG and then, if appropriate, a monitor hopefully paid for by your insurance, such as a ZIO® Patch, 24-hour Holter monitor, event recorder, or an MCOT.

- If you still can't figure it out, consider the shampoo approach— lather, rinse, repeat. There is no reason other than cost that you can't repeat a ZIO® Patch. Or, consider taking charge of your own diagnosis with something like the AliveCor Kardia™.

Here is a comparison of some of the various monitors mentioned above as well as estimated costs from an article I wrote in 2013.

	Continuous recording?	Duration	Real-time?	External electrodes and wires required?	Estimated Cost excludes placement and interpretation
Zio® Patch	Yes	Up to 14 days	No	No	$500
Heart Rate Monitors	No	Typically record for 10 seconds or less	Yes, rate only	No	Free to $300
AliveCor iPhone app	No	30 seconds	Yes	No	$75
Holter	Yes	Up to 2 days	No	Yes (3-6)	$250
Event Recorder	No	Up to 30 days	No	Varies (0-3)	$600
MCOT (Mobile Cardiac Outpatient Telemetry)	Yes	Up to 21 days	Yes	Yes (3)	$900

Figure 5.5: Cost comparison of heart rhythm monitoring devices.

Now, you know more about heart rhythm recordings than some doctors. Do you know what to call two orthopedic surgeons reading an EKG? A double-blind study.[5]

[5] Orthopedic surgeons are notoriously bad at reading EKGs.

6

How to save a life with CPR

Someone suffering sudden death from an arrhythmia will die without cardiopulmonary resuscitation (CPR). Anyone can do CPR without an official card from the Red Cross and you're better off trying than doing nothing.[1]

Here is what you need to do to perform CPR:

1. Shake the person who has collapsed to make sure the person is truly dying and not just "over served" from the local bar. Lie the patient flat on the floor on his or her back.

2. Have someone call 911 for emergency assistance (or if you are lucky, have someone bring an automatic external defibrillator (AED), which will talk you through what to do). If no one is around, CPR won't bring a person back to life, so if you can only do one thing, calling for an ambulance is the most important. Then, quickly return to the patient.

3. Begin CPR.

4. Press rhythmically on the person's chest. Press with the heel of your hand on the breast bone (firmly but not enough to break it) to the tune of "Stayin' Alive," the 1977 disco hit. If you do not know this awful Bee Gees song, do not look it up. Just press at a rate of about once a second. The American Heart Association instructs 80 times a minute but you aren't being graded here. Coincidentally, "Ah, ah, ah , ah, stayin' alive" is about 80 bpm.

5. Continue until help arrives.

[1] This said, I'd highly recommend the Red Cross (or other) trainings on CPR. The classes not only demonstrate the technique I'm about to describe but also will help you remain calm in a crisis situation.

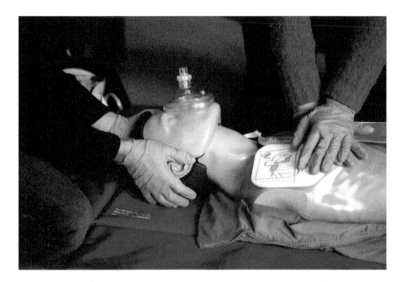

Figure 6.1: CPR being performed on a medical-training manikin (Photo by Rama/Wikimedia).

The newest research shows you no longer have to put your lips on the dying person and do mouth-to-mouth resuscitation. As sad as it is, people have died when bystanders have been afraid to touch their lips to the dying person because "I might get AIDS." For the record you can only get HIV from blood or sexual transmission. However, this newer CPR research has revealed that the "in with the good air" approach doesn't work very well because what we exhale doesn't have much oxygen, particularly for a dying person. The rhythmic chest compression is far more useful.

In recent years, AEDs like those you might see in an airport, have made an impact.[2] One large published study found that first-responder defibrillations occur in about 25% of out-of-hospital cardiac arrests now, nearly double that of just 5 years ago. As expected, prompt bystander CPR increases the chance of recovering without permanent brain injury. Survival rates have improved tremendously from the 6% they used to be:

- Waiting for EMS (paramedic) CPR and defibrillation, 10% survive

- CPR and bystander defibrillation (AED), survival rate 25%

- CPR, AED, then further EMT CPR and defibrillation, survival rate 33%

[2] Acronym reminder: AEDs = automatic external defibrillators.

Alec Momont, a grad student in the Netherlands, developed a prototype for an AED delivery by drone. After a call is placed to 911 (in Europe the emergency number is actually 112), the operator can determine the location by GPS and send a drone with an AED built-in, which has no traffic challenges and flies at 60 mph. At the scene, it lands and the 911 operator helps instruct the care through speakers and the drone's camera until paramedics arrive. Coming soon to a street corner near you.

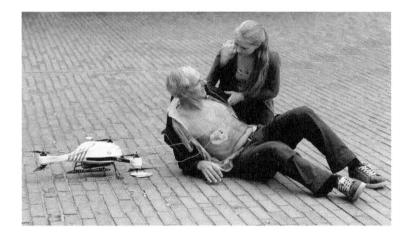

Figure 6.2: A drone-delivered defibrillator (With permission, Alec Momont, Delft University of Technology).

When someone goes into cardiac arrest, the first rule of thumb is to stay calm. This might be easier said than done but remember that the patient is the one with the disease. You cannot get hurt by doing CPR, but you could be a real hero if you keep your wits about you.[3]

Just do it and ignore the distracting thoughts, saving them for the TV interview later. The trick to surviving a stressful situation is to compartmentalize your thoughts and focus on the task at hand.

Admittedly, with all that adrenaline running through you, it is hard to stay calm. That is the real benefit of taking a CPR class, so that you will be familiar with the situation and stay calm.

Here is an unrelated story about managing stress. After 6 years of cardiac training in Colorado, I was moving with my brand-new bride to my first real job in La Jolla, California. I was driving a Ryder truck full of everything we owned (includ-

[3] The most common injuries sustained from CPR are rib fractures, with literature suggesting an incidence between 13% and 97%, and sternal fractures, with an incidence between 1% to 43%. While these injuries can require further intervention (assuming the patient survives the cardiac arrest), only 0.5% of them are life-threatening in their own right. A small price to pay for having your life saved.

ing all three of my shirts). At the very top of Vail Pass, just after one of those runaway truck turnouts, I pressed the brake pedal and it gave way. When I pushed the pedal, it just hit the floorboard without any braking. I called for my wife of 2 days to jump out because we weren't yet going very fast down I-70, a steep highway just above the town of Vail. She refused to jump out of the truck.

My first thought was panic, but then I remembered panic wouldn't do me any good.

I had my wife take the wheel while I knelt down under the dash to see what was wrong with the pedal. Imagine, handing the steering wheel to the passenger, sliding down on the floor board to check out the brake pedal as this massive truck careened down Vail Pass. Fortunately, I quickly figured out that the pedal had come disconnected from the lever that activates the hydraulic brakes. A 25-cent part (cotter pin) had broken! I used my hand to push the lever and the truck came to a halt, or I wouldn't be writing this book.

Now we still had to get into town to get it repaired. In my bride's purse, we found a wedding gift Cross pen and inserted it in place of the broken cotter pin. I pressed on the brake pedal but it broke too (not everything that works on MacGyver works in real life). So, I spent the next hour lying on the floor of the truck pushing the brake when instructed as we tediously drove into Vail to get it repaired. I attribute this survival story to my medical training where I learned to keep my wits at hospital cardiac arrests or Code Blues.

Remember the British war poster, "Keep calm and carry on?" When faced with a crisis, compartmentalize your thoughts. Focus on doing the CPR and the rest you can sort out later with a beer or two.[4]

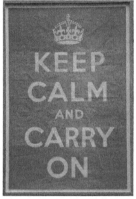

Figure 6.3: Original copy of the 1939 "Keep Calm And Carry On" poster (Image by UK government).

[4] The phone rings and the conversation starts, "Mom, don't be alarmed, I'm in the hospital!" She replies, "Son, after 4 years of med school, that joke is getting pretty old."

7
Arrhythmias 101: Slow and fast

In Chapter 2 we discussed the normal heart rhythm. Remember that we have 2.5 billion heartbeats in a typical lifetime. Thus, it is not surprising that not every beat is perfect. An occasional hiccup is no big deal but more serious arrhythmias affect the heart's ability to pump blood effectively and thus cause symptoms from sudden death to none at all (any of this sound familiar to you?)

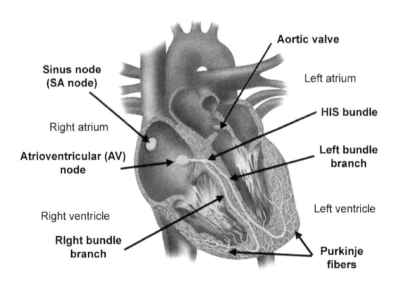

Figure 7.1: Cardiac conduction system (Modified from CEUFast.com with permission).

As a brief refresher, above is a wonderful picture of the normal heart's electrical system. Our heart rate is driven by the built-in pacemaker in the sinus (or sinoatrial) node. It then courses throughout the upper chambers (atria) through the

AV node to the pumping chambers (ventricles) through wires called bundle branches. So, how can this go wrong?

Arrhythmias come in many flavors. Just like in dating, our first concern is too slow or too fast?

7.1 Bradyarrhythmias ("slow" heart beats)

Doctors call slow heart beats *bradycardia* to sound superior because slow is too easy for you to understand. When we sleep, our pulse might dip into the 50s without a problem because you don't need very much blood carrying oxygen and nutrients pumped around to support your resting body. However, that same rate when you are running could make you faint. A heart rate in the 30s or slower, particularly associated with symptoms, such as fatigue, dizziness, or fainting, generally warrants treatment, like a pacemaker.

7.1.1 Sick sinus syndrome

Most commonly, abnormal bradycardia occurs from that upper built-in pacemaker, the sinus node, getting tired. We call this sinus node dysfunction or sick sinus syndrome, which is more fun to pronounce. While there are medicines that can temporarily increase the heart rate, none are safe to use long term. "No, doc, honest, I want that cocaine prescription only because I need it to speed my slow heart."

Symptoms and sinus node slowing often requires implanting a permanent pacemaker. An implanted pacemaker provides a reliable electrical signal to the heart to remind it to beat at the correct rate. The electrical output is too small to feel but is enough to trigger the heart to beat as it would from your own built-in sinus node pacemaker.

7.1.2 AV block

The second most common cause of slow heart rates is atrioventricular (AV) conduction disease. The normal AV node intentionally slows transmission of the electrical impulse from the atria to the ventricles. However, sometimes it gets too slow. We all love to classify things in threes but physicians still make it sound confusing. For AV block or skin burns, first degree is better than third degree. Unlike murder, where first degree is the worst, first-degree AV block is often a minor normal variant.

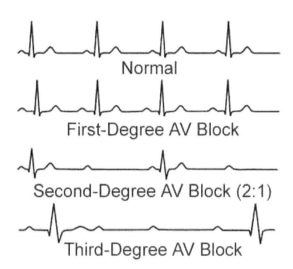

Figure 7.2: Degrees of AV block (Modified from MyKentuckyHeart.com with permission).

First-degree AV block is just a delay of the impulse longer than the normal 200 milliseconds (1/5th of a second) for each atrial beat. Often, there will be no symptoms.

Second-degree AV block is when the AV node doesn't let every atrial beat reach the ventricles. This too can be asymptomatic. However, if a pause exceeds 3 seconds that is typically long enough to be noticed. Pauses, whether from second- or third-degree AV block of 3 seconds or more, particularly when associated with symptoms, are a good reason for a pacemaker.[1]

Now for another quiz question. What do you think the best treatment is for third-degree AV block? Correct—a permanent pacemaker. These days, implanted pacemakers come in several varieties, with one, two, or three leads and even the newest without any leads. Chapter 12 covers pacemakers in detail.

[1] At least once a month, I see a patient complaining of not feeling quite right who ends up having third-degree or complete AV block! They are kept alive by their backup natural pacemakers at 30 or 40 beats per minute.

7.1.3   Bundle branch block (BBB)

I've covered slow rhythms from the sinus and AV nodes, but there are other common conduction issues that can cause slowing.

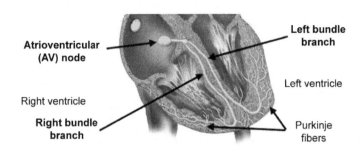

Atrioventricular (AV) node

Left bundle branch

Right ventricle

Left ventricle

Right bundle branch

Purkinje fibers

Figure 7.3: Bundle branches extending below the AV node (Modified from CEU-Fast.com with permission).

Bundle branch block is another alliterative medical term, like sick sinus syndrome or dead as a door nail. Two bundle branches extend below the AV node, the right and the left, with the latter sometimes subdivided into the left anterior and left posterior fascicles.

These bundle branches allow rapid electrical conduction to the bottom of the heart so that muscle contraction happens bottom to top to squirt blood out the major vessels, such as the aorta. Think of the bundle branches as just electrical wires that transmit the electricity to the bottom of the heart so that it beats first and pumps blood up and out to the body.

Commonly, one of these bundles can stop working, from age, disease, calcification, trauma, and so on. Fortunately, many of our organs are redundant, such as two kidneys, so you can often get by fine if you have just one bundle branch blocked.

An electrocardiogram (EKG) will tell you whether you have right or left BBB. If you have BBB and feel fine, no treatment is usually needed. Nevertheless, it is a good thing to know in case you show up in an ER someday and a doctor asks if this condition is old or new. Unless your EKG is absolutely normal, you should keep a copy on you, either as a photograph stored on your phone, or get a copy for your home medical file and your wallet/purse. Something as simple as BBB can buy you a night in the hospital when you show up in an ER after a minor car accident and no one knows if it's new or old.

Cookies make everything easier to understand. The figure shown comes from a dentist who teaches EKGs and likes to bake. I like her marketing approach—cookies cause cavities and dentists treat cavities. I guess I should start passing out cigarettes on the street corner.

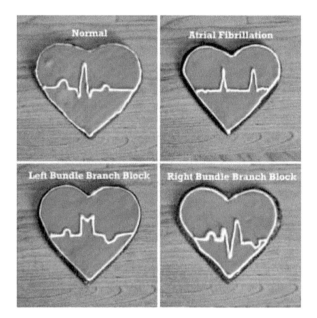

Figure 7.4: Cookie hearts showing bundle branch block (With permission, Erica Pitera, DMD, EricaSweetTooth.com)

Now when one of the bundle branches is blocked and the electricity in your heart has to take a detour, there might be an issue. As the electrical conduction to the pumping chambers (ventricles) slows, that can lead to poor heart pumping. Blockage of two of the three major branches, called bifascicular block, is even a little worse. Nevertheless, BBB is most commonly asymptomatic and something you can live with safely for decades. However, if both bundle branches fail, just like what happens when both kidneys conk out, you have a problem. The treatment is, you guessed it, a pacemaker.

Before you figure out that cardiology is too simple and you don't need me, let's move on.

7.2   Tachyarrhythmias ("fast" heart rhythms)

Physicians use the prefix "tachy" not for the loud clothes we wear on the golf course but for "fast." This term fits with rule number one from the first day of medical school, "Medical words must be longer than normal words."

Similar to bradyarrhythmias, there is no magic high number that makes tachycardia always bad. Even a 50 year old running for a bus can get his heart rate briefly to 150 bpm or more. However, any rate more than 120, not from normal sinus rhythm (called sinus tachycardia) is generally considered abnormal.

Tachycardia rhythms can be divided into *regular* or *irregular*. This distinction has nothing to do with your bowel habits. Regular refers to the steady "beat-beat-beat" like a good drummer. You can predict when the next beat is due. Try feeling your own pulse at your wrist now to understand what regular rhythm is about.

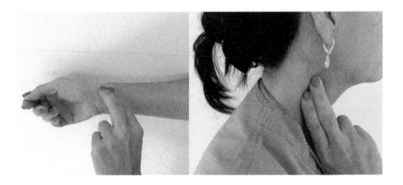

Figure 7.5: A pretty EP nurse (she made me write that) demonstrates how to check your own pulse. The left panel shows the radial pulse, easiest to feel. The right panel shows the carotid pulse. It's closer to the heart so more accurate if your rhythm is irregular. Figure out the rate in 1-minute (measure 15 seconds and multiply by 4).

Irregular rhythms come in two varieties. Infrequent or *regularly irregular* pulses can be from a single early beat. You might feel beat-beat-early beat-short pause-beat-beat. These isolated early beats can be normal and often are not even felt. In those who do feel them, typically they don't actually feel the early beat but the pause after resulting in an extra-strong next normal beat. The early beat is usually associated with the heart filling poorly with blood but for the next normal beat, it allows the heart to fill a little longer. This "whoosh" from the super-normal beat after the pause is actually what is sensed as a brief palpitation. That is why these early beats are also called skipped beats, though actually they are not skipped, just sometimes too early to feel. By definition, these isolated early beats cause palpitations that last no longer than a second or two.

Early beats from the upper chambers used to be just called PACs, premature atrial contractions, to go along with PVCs, premature ventricular contractions. But, no, that made it too

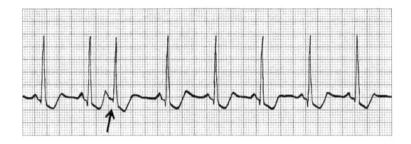

Figure 7.6: A single, iso-lated, premature atrial beat, also called an SVE, supraventricular ectopic. A mild pause follows the early beat, which is of-ten more easily felt when checking your pulse.

easy for laypeople to understand so now physicians call these early upper-chamber beats SVEs, which stands for supraven-tricular ectopics. That occurred when we learned that some PACs don't actually originate in the "atria" but in the AV node junction region, hence the need to drop "atria" and substitute "supraventricular" (meaning above the ventricles). Ectopic sounds more complicated, than contraction so that was changed too.[2] Anyway, if you want to impress an EP doctor (and I am sure that is high on your bucket list), use SVE instead of PAC.

[2] Ectopic means from an abnormal location.

As mentioned, we all have SVEs several times every day. However, these beats can be the trigger for other arrhythmias, such as AF and sustained supraventricular tachycardia (SVT). Or, they can be perfectly normal.

A long-time EP colleague and pioneer, Eric Prystowsky (note his initials; he was destined from birth to be an EP doc) taught me the concept that an SVE is like turning your starter in your car. If you have no engine, it cannot cause the motor to run. However, an SVE can be the trigger for a sustained arrhythmia only in those who also have a substrate for an arrhythmia, in this analogy, an engine. Thus, an SVE will cause the engine to run (that is, heart racing, such as SVT) when there is a second pathway or some other problem. Frequently, people who have sustained heart racing that starts with an SVE get frightened when they still feel these single early beats after a successful treatment, such as an ablation. However, the motor will never run if the engine is removed.[3]

[3] It is nearly impossible to entirely eliminate SVEs either with medicine or ablation, so, in general, don't worry about them.

The other type of irregular fast rhythm is described as irreg-ularly irregular. I know this again sounds like Donald Rums-feld's "unknown unknowns," but there is a method to this madness. If the next beat's timing is totally unpredictable, that is not only irregular but irregularly irregular. Imagine a drummer on drugs, or is that redundant?

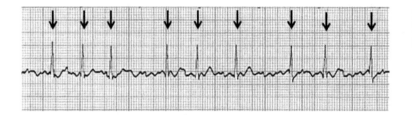

Figure 7.7: AF, an irregularly irregular rhythm, at 90 bpm.

The figure above shows how the most common irregularly irregular rhythm, AF, must feel to a patient. Check out the arrows and see how you cannot predict when the next beat will occur.

Similarly, when you check your pulse in AF, you never know when the next beat will occur. To complicate this further, these rhythms can be slow, normal, or fast in rate, even though they are irregular. To reiterate, rhythm refers to the regularity of the heart, rate to the actual number of beats over time.

7.3 Supraventricular tachycardias (SVTs)

Regular rapid rhythms from the upper part of the heart are called SVTs.[4]

SVTs come is in several flavors:

[4] Remember, *supraventricular* means originating at or above the AV node.

- Inappropriate sinus tachycardia (IST)

- Paroxysmal atrial tachycardia (PAT)

- Paroxysmal supraventricular tachycardia (PSVT)

  – AV node reentry

  – Wolff-Parkinson-White (WPW) syndrome and its variants

- Atrial flutter

- Atrial fibrillation (AF)

7.3.1 Inappropriate sinus tachycardia (IST)

IST is sinus tachycardia (fast normal rhythm) that is not appropriate for the circumstances. Remember, that sinus tachycardia is the term we use for rapid racing of the heart driven from the normal sinus node—for instance, every time we run or climb stairs.

IST occurs when the heart races from an overactive or diseased sinus node for no good reason. Thus, to make this diagnosis, you must exclude activity (usually, not very tough), fever, drugs, anxiety, or other hidden illness, such as an overactive thyroid. Wearing a long-term monitor, IST patients might have sudden rapid sinus rates to 140 bpm or more even when sound asleep and relaxed. Unfortunately, patients with anxiety, such as panic attacks, can be misdiagnosed as having an arrhythmia like IST. Actually, it is far more common for the opposite. Patients who have IST, as well as other arrhythmias, might be told they are having panic attacks when, in fact, they might have a treatable arrhythmia that made them anxious. I have witnessed many "crazy" people who became normal after their arrhythmia was fixed.[5]

[5] How do crazy people travel through the woods? They take the psychopath.

7.3.2   Paroxysmal atrial tachycardia (PAT)

Paroxysmal atrial tachycardia is both an old and new term. It used to be the term that docs used for all SVTs.

Today, atrial tachycardia is actually a specific term for a type of regular supraventricular tachycardia that arises from diseased areas of the atria separate from the sinus node or AV node areas. Atrial tachycardias can be very difficult to treat because they occur randomly and cannot always be triggered in a catheter electrophysiology study. It is often caused by abnormal cells called ectopic sites that fire arbitrarily.

This can give EP docs headaches when you have the ablation catheters in place and you can't find the site of the PAT.

If doctors use the term AT or PAT and are over 60 and not specialists, they mean any upper chamber arrhythmia like SVT. If your doctor needs a beard or glasses to look older, he probably means that PAT is the more modern usage of a focal atrial area for the rhythm problem.

7.3.3   Paroxysmal supraventricular tachycardia (PSVT)

PSVT also has several names.   Paroxysmal means it comes and goes but because PSVT is almost never stuck fast permanently, many just use the term SVT. In general, EP doctors use the term SVT as a grab bag phrase for all regular, fast upper-chamber arrhythmias lumped together. Confusing? Yes, this is intentional.

Typical PSVT is actually the coolest and easiest to diagnose and cure. As opposed to isolated wild heart cells of atrial tachycardia, an abnormal pathway causes PSVT. In the normal heart, we discussed the normal pathways from the AV node to the ventricles. Think of these as electrical wires in our hearts. If you have more than one wire (pathway) in your heart, then it is possible for the heart to conduct down one pathway and up the other, round and round. Patients with PSVT have an extra pathway that is usually silent most of the time, adjacent to the normal AV node and conducting normally right alongside it. This problem is called a dual AV nodal pathways.

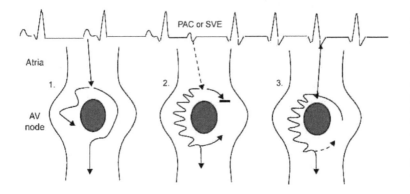

Figure 7.8: 1. A normal beat travels down both AV node pathways. 2. An early beat (SVE) blocks down one and travels slowly down the second pathway. 3. This second pathway allows the electrical current to travel back up the blocked pathway, initiating a reentrant tachycardia (Modified from C.Pappone, AF-ablation.org with permission).

As shown in the drawing, if a single early beat, a common SVE, arrives at just the right time, it might not be able to travel down both of these parallel pathways. If the heart tissue below is activated and finds the extra pathway doing nothing, it may conduct backwards right up through it, as the dashed line shows. This then becomes like a dog chasing its tail, the conduction continues in a circle within the AV node. Hence the name, AV node reentrant tachycardia (AVNRT), more commonly called PSVT. Typically, PSVT is 140 to 200 bpm and overrides the rest of the heart. It might continue indefinitely until treated.

Patients with PSVT might feel the trigger (the engine's starter) but then they feel a sudden, rapid regular racing of their heart that doesn't stop for minutes or longer. Depending

on the rate, age, and associated problems, PSVT can cause fainting or severe near-fainting sensations. Imagine how you would
feel if your heart rate jumps from 60 to 200 and gets stuck there;
the pump becomes less efficient, the blood pressure drops, and
there you go, swooning to the ground.[6] Often, patients who
have this get it repeatedly every few weeks or months. Some
are provoked by certain things from exercise to bending over
to stimulants like espresso. Thus, med school rule number four
applies here, "If it hurts when you do that, don't do that."

Sometimes, patients learn to terminate the PSVT by doing
a trick called a *vagal maneuver*. The AV node can be affected
by external inputs from the brain, particularly through the
parasympathetic nerves, the one to the heart is the vagus nerve.
So, if you do a vagal maneuver you can make the PSVT stop
immediately through activation of these nerve inputs. It is
important to learn how to properly do a vagal maneuver from
a physician because there is a mild risk, particularly if not
performed while lying down.

Common vagal maneuvers include:

- Valsalva (forced exhale against a closed airway, like when
  you are bearing down)

- Carotid sinus massage (intentional massage of the neck
  artery on one side)

- Diving reflex (immersing your face in ice cold water, yes
  really)

- Gagging (the ice water doesn't seem so bad now, does it?)

The Airman shown holding his nose and straining illustrates
how to do a Valsalva maneuver, often the best of the vagal
maneuvers to terminate PSVT. If these vagal tricks don't work,
PSVT often continues indefinitely, so a prompt trip to the ER is
necessary (don't drive yourself).

In earlier days, PSVT might have required a long wait followed by medicines that didn't work well or even an external
shock called a cardioversion to get the heart back to normal.

Today, there is a long wait for your insurance to be checked
followed by a fast acting intravenous medicine, adenosine, that
stops the racing. While adenosine stops the heart for a second

[6] Terms like swooning and consumption were more common in Victorian times. Swooning is fainting, most commonly from a serious heart problem, not just being in love. Consumption was a fatal lung disease discovered to be TB, which is now mostly eradicated in the United States, though we all still have to get annual skin tests as medical professionals. Consumption (TB) really killed Chopin, Orwell, and Chekov (not the one on *Star Trek*).

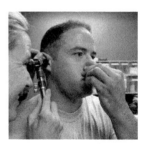

Figure 7.9: Patient demonstrating a Valsalva maneuver. Apparently, the doctor
was also worried that he'd
blow his brains out his ear
(Photo by U.S. Air Force
Airman 1st Class Kate
Thornton/Wikimedia).

or 2, and might make you feel light-headed, it will reliably and safely terminate PSVT. Unfortunately, there is no oral version (and there never will be because your heart really does stop for a short time).

PSVT can be treated with daily medications but that is often the second choice today. Daily medicines don't work that well, have side effects, and are difficult to remember to take for a problem that happens infrequently.

Catheter ablation has become the standard of care for PSVT and is generally recommended even after just one episode. Ablation for PSVT usually is a one-time procedure curing this problem in about 95% of cases; the accessory pathway or "extra wire" is eliminated with heat from the ablation catheter leaving the normal AV node pathway intact. This type of ablation essentially returns the heart's electrical system back to normal.

7.3.4   Wolff-Parkinson-White (WPW) syndrome

Called WPW, Wolff-Parkinson-White syndrome is even more interesting than common PSVT. Although rare (less than 1 in 1,000 people), WPW is very helpful in teaching us how arrhythmias work. First of all, you need to learn why it is called Wolff-Parkinson-White. This syndrome was named after three ancient (defined as older than me) cardiologists who met each other only once in 1930. Fortunately, they stood in order for their selfie photo. Back then, I guess iPhones could only take pictures in black and white.

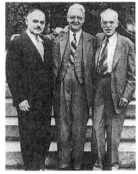

Figure 7.10: From left to right, Doctors Wolff, Parkinson, and White (Photo courtesy Heart Rhythm Society Archives).

You might recall that I mentioned the only way for the heart's electrical activity to get from the atria to the ventricles was through the AV node. I lied. There actually are conditions when there is a second pathway from the atria to the ventricles, separate from the AV node. Rarely, when the heart is developing in the womb, extra tissue might remain behind forming an electrical connection between the upper and lower chambers. So when the heart beats, a beat might start like normal in the sinus node and travel throughout the atria. However, it then has a choice of going down the normal AV node or down this extra wire, called an accessory pathway. As a result, the resting EKG is abnormal, called pre-excited. I'm not so sure about that term because the heart is either excited or it isn't, but the term remains.

A typical WPW pattern is seen on every single beat of an EKG with a special early deflection called the *delta wave*. I have no idea why these guys chose that term because it is between the P wave and QRS complex. Hey, guys, why not PQ wave?[7]

When you have two pathways, just like PSVT above, the situation can arise that a premature beat goes down only one wire and not the other. Thus, you have the classic setup for a reentrant tachycardia, most commonly down the normal AV node and back up the accessory pathway wherever it is located. These accessory pathways of WPW syndrome can connect the atria and ventricles anywhere around the two AV valves, the tricuspid and mitral, separate from the normal AV node connection. Nearly identical to PSVT, this presents the possibility of a rapid upper-chamber racing that can be terminated with the Valsalva maneuver or with the medicine adenosine.

[7] By the way, do you know what you call an EKG of someone with a rapid rate and a low blood potassium? "P on U syndrome." Yuk, yuk. You see, low potassium makes something called a U wave prominent (after P and QRS comes U) and the next P wave rides on top of it. P on U, get it? We EP docs are hilarious; just you wait.

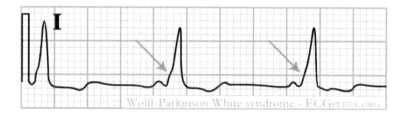

Figure 7.11: WPW can be seen on every heartbeat as a delta wave between the P and Q (With permission, ECGpedia.org).

To make it even more complex, sometimes the extra pathway is concealed so that it isn't evident on a regular EKG, only working in the backwards (ventricle to atrium) direction. Thus, when an EP doctor does a routine PSVT ablation, the doc always needs to look for this rare congenital variant. Fortunately, today WPW can be consistently cured in about 95% of cases.[8]

The history of WPW syndrome treatment is fascinating. Before open heart surgery, doctors used medicine like digoxin, formulated from the foxglove plant. It actually could make WPW worse and led to some episodes of sudden death. Without medication, about 1 in 100 to 500 WPW patients are at risk for sudden death from a rare problem called atrio-ventricular fibrillation (believe me, you don't want to catch that). Regular atrial fibrillation travels down the accessory pathway without the natural slowing properties of the AV node and can aggra-

[8] Because today WPW can be easily diagnosed by a regular EKG and reliably ablated, someone wrote a clever editorial a few years ago "The Wolff is an endangered species." I told you that EP doctors are hilarious, didn't I?

vate the ventricles into fibrillating.

In the 1970s, after open heart surgery was figured out, Duke University physicians John Gallagher and Jimmy Cox, cardiologist and cardiac surgeon respectively, masterfully discovered a way to cure WPW syndrome. They mapped the beating heart during an open chest procedure, figured out which quadrant the WPW pathway resided, and then placed the patient on cardiopulmonary bypass to fix it. Because the pathways are invisible to the eye, Dr. Cox would actually separate the atrium from the ventricle in the location mapped and then suture it back onto the ventricle. Amazingly, it worked quite well and their pioneering work helped create the field of cardiac EP. Of course, today, WPW syndrome is cured with an ablation through catheters in a vein. Patients are often home by dinner, cured for life.[9]

In the mid-1980s, this open heart arrhythmia surgery was done at only a select few hospitals in the world. In 1986, I referred a patient from Scripps to Stanford and flew up to watch the case. One of my Scripps heart surgeon associates, Sam Keeley, got wind and joined me. Fortunately, Sam had trained at Duke under Dr. Cox. At Stanford, we observed a successful operation. More importantly, we realized how primitive this operation was at the time and copied the Stanford setup at our community hospital, performing the first open heart arrhythmia surgery in southern California at Scripps in 1987.

[9] Did you know that open heart surgery was first done before the advent of the heart-lung bypass machine? Children with a hole in their heart would have their blood shunted to a parent (with the same blood type) on an adjacent OR table, allowing the child's heart to be stopped for surgery, keeping them alive while a surgeon quickly sewed the hole shut and restarted the heart.

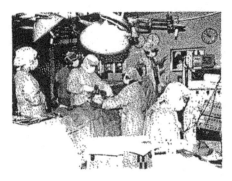

Figure 7.12: The early days of arrhythmia surgery. Dr. Keeley is operating while Dr. Higgins is interpreting recorded signals from the open heart. Apparently, this was so long ago that we only had grainy black and white photos (Arrhythmia surgery in a community hospital, *Cardio*, 1989).

In those days, we had no device support and bought electrical parts and tools (even a Craftsman screwdriver), sterilized them, and used them during surgery. Because you could justify the risks of surgery for only the sickest patients, it was amazing to wake them up and find the EKG had become normal, a true cure. With destruction of the accessory pathway, the EKG's extra delta wave also resolves.

Initially, we performed single point-to-point mapping directly on the beating heart through the open chest using a hand-held probe. Amazingly, we performed 47 arrhythmia surgery procedures in the first 18 months yet had no perioperative deaths, a remarkable accomplishment for the time. It is extraordinary to think that such innovation would never be allowed today with all the government restrictions on research, albeit generally for valid reasons. Nevertheless, the treatment of life-threatening arrhythmias moved quickly in this unregulated era (we did have hospital Investigational Review Board permission) and many patients were helped and survived.

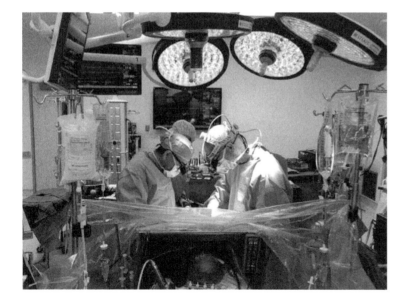

Figure 7.13: Open heart surgery today, little has changed other than better photography.

This type of pioneering open heart surgery for WPW syndrome taught us budding "electrical cardiologists" how reentrant arrhythmias worked and formed the basis for the modern catheter-based approach to treating WPW, PSVT, and a host of other arrhythmias. As someone famous once said, "You must walk on the shoulders of giants before you can run."

7.3.5   Atrial flutter

Heart flutters is another old term used for that feeling just
before you swoon. People who feel a fluttering in their chest
could have any arrhythmia because it is essentially a synonym
for palpitations. However, *atrial flutter* is an entirely different
animal. It too is a reentrant arrhythmia.

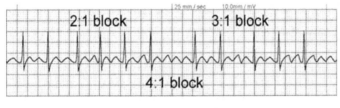

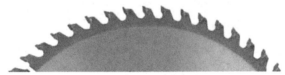

Figure 7.14: Typical atrial
flutter with variable block
compared to a real saw's
teeth.

In atrial flutter, the atria beats regularly but very fast, at 240
to 340 bpm. Thanks to that smart AV node we all received at
birth, these beats don't all get to the ventricles (generally, if
your ventricles beat more than 250 bpm, your heart gives out
and you quickly die). These impulses are allowed through
the AV node in an alternating fashion. Most commonly, atrial
flutter occurs in the atrium at about 300 bpm with 2:1 block,
so the ventricle goes at 150 bpm. If you are on medication,
the degree of block might be greater. The same atrial flutter at
300 bpm with 4:1 block would result in a pulse of 75 because
only every fourth beat gets to the ventricles. Sometimes, it isn't
regular with alternating levels of block as shown.

Depending on the EKG lead, atrial flutter gives a classic
"saw-tooth" appearance because the smaller waves are perfectly
regular. Like everything in medicine, there is typical atrial flutter and atypical, so it actually doesn't have to be saw-toothed or
even regular to be atrial flutter.

It is important to realize that, although related, atrial flutter
is much different from atrial fibrillation (AF). Only about 20
years ago, some EP doctors far smarter than me first recognized
that flutter occurs from a very large reentrant circuit. As shown

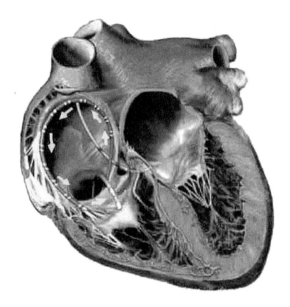

Figure 7.15: Atrial flutter counter-clockwise reentrant circuit. Note the ablation catheter in the cavotricuspid isthmus where the circuit is eliminated (Modified from Blaufus Multimedia with permission).

in yellow, the circuit of atrial flutter travels around both atria at 300 bpm (about 75 miles an hour!) in a huge loop.

Amazingly, for this loop to persist, it must travel through a small area in the lower-right atrium called the cavotricuspid isthmus (CTI). If you ablate a small line, about 1/2 inch long destroying the ability to conduct electricity between two electrically silent structures, atrial flutter will disappear for good.[10]

7.3.6   Atrial fibrillation

AF is the most common serious arrhythmia. If you are old school, you call it "A Fib," but if you are younger and hip (you need glasses or a beard to look like a doctor), it is "AF." Of course, that makes no sense because atrial flutter starts with an A and F too.

AF is a complex arrhythmia, which on an EKG is irregularly irregular, so you can't predict the next beat. In the untreated heart, the AV node is bombarded with impulses even faster than flutter at 450 to 600 bpm commonly translating to a ventricular rate (pulse rate) of 120 to 150 bpm. In addition to being irregular, it is too fast, unless you are on medication or have a lazy AV node. AF is the bane of my existence because it causes

[10] The inferior vena cava is the giant vein bringing all the blood from the lower body back to the right heart. The tricuspid valve is the large valve between these two chambers. Hence the cavotricuspid isthmus is the space between the two. These two anatomic structures are electrically silent so by extending the CTI line here, the atrial flutter reentry is routinely cured for good.

more symptoms, is hard to cure even with ablation, and is a common cause of strokes. AF is discussed in more detail in Chapter 16.

7.4   Ventricular tachyarrhythmias

So far we've covered slow rhythms, bradyarrhythmias, and tachycardias from the upper chambers, now we get to the really bad ones.

Ventricular tachyarrhythmias, rapid rhythm from the lower pumping chambers, essentially only come in two flavors, bad (VT) and worse (VF).

7.4.1   Ventricular tachycardia (VT)

VT is regular, rapid racing of the lower chambers. Even though this rhythm is regular (beat-beat-beat), it is often fast enough that the blood flow out of the heart is so poor it causes fainting (syncope).

We faint from VT for a host of reasons in addition to the rapid rate. First of all, the upper chambers are electronically disconnected so we lose the atrial kick of regular rhythm. Secondly, the disorganized origin of VT might begin anywhere in the lower chambers, so even if organized, the pumping of blood is less effective than the same rate in a sinus rhythm. Finally, if that isn't bad enough, VT often degenerates into VF and causes sudden death.

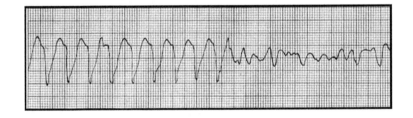

Figure 7.16: Ventricular tachycardia (VT) degenerating into ventricular fibrillation (VF), from bad to worse.

7.4.1.1   Ischemic VT

VT comes in two major varieties, ischemic and non-ischemic. Ischemic VT is associated with a prior heart attack. Remember how I explained earlier that a heart attack is a blocked blood vessel to the heart and is not the same as sudden death? Well, if you survive this blockage, it still causes scarring in your heart if blood flow isn't reestablished within minutes. With time, this can lead to heart failure and, unfortunately, sudden death, often years later. Most commonly, only massive heart attacks or multiple ones create enough scarring to cause VT. Amazingly, VT is also caused by a reentrant pathway that develops around the scar.

One of the most important medical research studies of the last few decades (I don't say that just because I was on the executive committee) was called MADIT (Multicenter Automatic Defibrillator Implantation Trial). MADIT (pronounced like "made-it" not "mad-it") randomized people with a prior big heart attack, some to receive an implanted defibrillator and the others to get what in the 1990s was "conventional treatment," medications or nothing.

If you had a weakened heart muscle from prior heart attack(s), the chance of dying was more than 50% by 5 years, a worse risk than most cancers. Receiving an implanted defibrillator cuts the death rate by nearly one half!

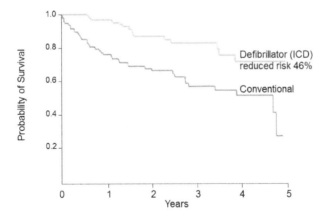

Figure 7.17: MADIT study compared the best conventional treatment to preventive therapy with an implanted defibrillator. Mortality with conventional treatment exceeded 50% at 5 years. (With permission, *New England Journal of Medicine*).

The MADIT investigators recognized that a prior heart attack resulting in a weakened heart muscle had a tremendous risk of sudden death.

A simple echocardiogram can determine your ejection fraction (EF). This is the single most important predictor of death

from heart disease, far better than cholesterol or weight. A normal EF is about 60% meaning that a normal heart pumps out
about 60% of the blood with each beat because the ventricle
doesn't empty entirely. The criteria for the first MADIT study
was an EF below 35% and MADIT II, 30%. Thus, if your EF is
that low, you have a greater risk of sudden death from VT and
VF.

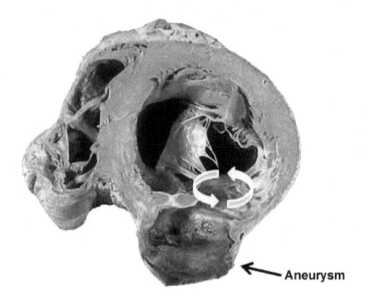

Aneurysm

Figure 7.18: Autopsy
specimen of a heart with
a thinned area called
an aneurysm, scarred
from prior heart attack.
The border areas of this
scar cause reentrant VT
which led to sudden death.
(With permission, Medical
Library, University of Utah).

Back to ischemic VT. The heart autopsy shown illustrates the
scarring of the ventricle that allowed a reentrant arrhythmia
to develop. Treatment options, outlined elsewhere, include
ablation (generally reserved for slower VTs), drugs (really don't
help much and have mostly been abandoned now for VT), and
an implanted defibrillator. Although it seems a bit simplistic
to choose a treatment that responds to a problem after it starts,
as opposed to trying to prevent it altogether, the implantable
cardioverter defibrillator (ICD) has saved more lives than just
about any modern medical advance.

7.4.1.2   Nonischemic VT

Nonischemic VT also usually happens in weak hearts. These
heart problems are called *nonischemic cardiomyopathies*. That
translates exactly (well almost) from the Latin "heart mus-

cle disease not from a heart attack." Nonischemic cardiomyopathies can be caused by:

- Infection, usually viral (a really bad chest cold possibly years ago)

- Genetic problems, such as hypertrophic cardiomyopathy

- Alcoholism (remember what mom said, everything in moderation)

- Medications, especially certain cancer drugs (I've got good news and bad news...)

- Prolonged tachycardia from any cause

- Pacing the right ventricle alone (causes the heart to beat out of synch)

- Rare postpartum complications due to pregnancy

- Rare issues from spider bites to HIV to Chagas disease and others

The most common cause of nonischemic cardiomyopathy is idiopathic, which is Latin for "Doctors don't know the cause but want to sound smart so they make up big words."

In the United States, about 70% of cardiomyopathies are from heart attacks, the remaining 30% are nonischemic. In other countries that ratio varies tremendously, about 50/50 in Europe. In Latin America, Chagas disease alone is the most common cause of cardiomyopathy. Chagas disease is a parasite that eats the heart and is transmitted through a bug bite (this section brought to you by the Latin American Tourism Bureau). Any cardiomyopathy can cause VT or sudden death. And the treatment, for those who are taking the advanced test is, yup, an implanted defibrillator, an ICD.

7.4.2   *Ventricular fibrillation (VF)*

Saving the worst for last, we get to ventricular fibrillation or VF. Ancient Egyptians as far back as 1500 BC (some say 3500 BC) described VF as:

If the heart trembles, has little power, and sinks, the disease is advanced and death is near.

These Egyptians must have been time travelers, confirmed by the fact this quote is in English. Our knowledge and treatment didn't progress beyond that understanding until about 100 years ago, more than 5,000 years later. Amazingly, it wasn't until the mid 1950s that a bright Harvard cardiologist, Bernard Lown, popularized that heart disease and sudden cardiac death might be reversible and survivable. Until then, heart attacks and heart failure were treated primarily with strict bed rest. The controversial Dr. Lown amazingly recommended that patients get out of bed, heresy at the time. Back then, the short-term death rate from a heart attack was more than 35%, partly due to blood clots from the legs traveling to the heart and lungs from the prolonged bed rest.

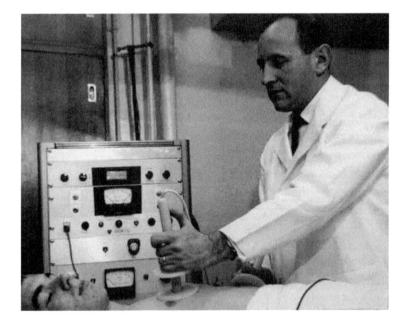

Figure 7.19: Dr. Bernard Lown demonstrating the first defibrillator, undoubtedly on a med student "volunteer"(Photo courtesy Heart Rhythm Society Archives).

Next, Dr. Lown, with the help of an electrical engineer, experimented with electricity applied directly to the heart. They first tried alternating current (similar to power from an electrical outlet) and found it *caused* VF. I believe his famous quote was, "I hate it when that happens."

Finally, in 1961, Dr. Lown tried direct current (one-way flow of electricity) applied quickly and directly to the heart. It converted VF to a normal rhythm in animals, so he tried it with people. Dr. Lown told the first patient it was untried therapy but "in a few hours you will be dead" without it. The hospital objected, but Dr. Lown said he would accept full responsibility; back then this approach was good enough. Fortunately, the first patient survived and was discharged a day later. Compare this to informed consent, investigational review boards, the Food and Drug Administration, and other regulations we have today.

It is difficult to estimate how many lives have been saved by Dr. Lown's invention. Even heart surgeons quickly caught on. They used alternating current to intentionally cause VF, stopping the heart so they could operate quickly to fix a structural problem, and then used direct current to start it up again. I repeat, this incredible device has saved many lives.

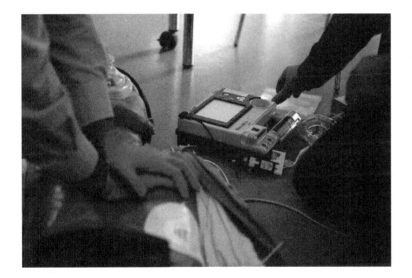

Figure 7.20: Paramedics ready a modern defibrillator during training (Photo by Rama/Wikimedia).

Dr. Lown wasn't perfect. In 1972, he was highly critical of the concept of the then investigational implantable cardioverter defibrillator, delaying its acceptance. He invented the external defibrillator but was dead-set against the internal defibrillator. A famous editorial of his in the American Heart Association's premier journal *Circulation* stated, "the implanted defibrillator represents an imperfect solution in search of a plausible and practical application."

Today, the ICD is routine with more than 100,000 implanted every year in the U.S. alone. Oh well, you can't win 'em all. Perhaps Dr. Lown didn't like the fact that the implantable defibrillator was developed at rival Johns Hopkins rather than Harvard. Still, we owe Dr. Lown and those first defibrillator patients a big *thank you*!

7.5   Wrap

It is reasonable to approach heart rhythms with an algorithm. I must mention my disclaimer again. You should not be your own doctor.[11]

This algorithm is for general education purposes only to help you understand the different types of arrhythmias:

1. Heart rate during arrhythmia:

    (a) 60 to 100 at rest, normal range

    (b) Less than 60, bradycardia

    (c) More than 100, tachycardia of some type

2. Is it regular or irregular?

    (a) If normal rate and regular rhythm, you probably don't need an EP doc.

    (b) If isolated irregular beats and normal rate, it's probably SVEs or PVCs, quantitate.[12]

       i. If more than 5,000 to 10,000 a day, see an EP doc.

       ii. If less than 500 a day, ignore.

       iii. In between 500 to 5,000, it might still be best to ignore before trying medication.

    (c) If it's irregular, sustained and fast, it's probably AF, document.

    (d) If it's irregular and normal rate, document because it could be slower AF.

    (e) If it's regular and fast, you need an EKG during rhythm.

       i. If it's narrow and fast, it is some type of SVT.

       ii. If it's wide, it might be VT or SVT with something unusual like a bundle branch block too.

[11] Remember the old line, "The doctor who treats himself has a fool for a patient."

[12] Remember, an SVE is a supraventricular ectopic where "ectopic" means out of place. A PVC is a premature ventricular contraction.

Here comes the final exam for Arrhythmias 101. How do you treat sudden death or VF?

If you answered an implanted defibrillator, you pass and can go on to the next chapter![13]

[13] Remember that the more technical term for an implanted defibrillator is an *implantable cardioverter defibrillator (ICD)*.

"Slow" heart rhythms (bradycardia)		"Fast" heart rhythms (tachycardia)
Sick sinus syndrome AV block Bundle branch block	**Above the AV node - supraventricular techycardias (SVTS)**	Inappropriate sinus tachycardia Paroxysmal supraventricular tachycardia (PSVT) - AV node reentry - Wolff-Parkinson-White syndrome and its variants Atrial flutter Paroxysmal atrial tachycardia (PAT) Isolated SVEs or PVCs Atrial fibrillation (AF)
	Below the AV node (ventricular)	Ventricular tachycardia (VT) - Ischemic - Non-ischemic Ventricular fibrillation (VF)

Table 7.1: Summary of slow and fast arrhythmias.

8
Risk factors

Everyone likes to know their risk of having a problem, particularly those that are potentially reversible. Now, if we all had the willpower to do something about it, cardiologists would have more time for golf.

8.1   Heart attack and coronary artery disease factors

This book is about arrhythmias in particular, but the risk factors for developing a heart attack are understood best and worth reviewing. First of all, for purposes of these risk factors, the risks are identical when discussing heart attack (also called myocardial infarction) or for developing coronary artery disease (CAD).

As you know, the heart is a muscle, different from your peripheral (skeletal) muscles because it beats continuously. Thus, this cardiac muscle is particularly dependent on receiving continuous oxygen and nutrients. You can have a "leg attack" when there is permanent loss of blood flow to a leg muscle and never even know it. The peripheral muscles have a better ability to receive blood flow from multiple sources, called collaterals. Amazingly, the heart and brain, our two most important organs have inadequate collateral arteries, so when a major one gets blocked, problems happen.

CAD is the process of your heart arteries narrowing, restricting blood flow.

Cardiologists used to think this was due to a plaque of cholesterol, which gradually increased, narrowing the artery just like a clogged pipe until it eventually blocked causing a complete loss of oxygen to the selected area and, thus, a heart attack. We now know this situation is rarely true. The plaque remains part of the problem; it actually looks like a hardened yellow overcooked egg yolk.

Normal Artery   Narrowing of Artery

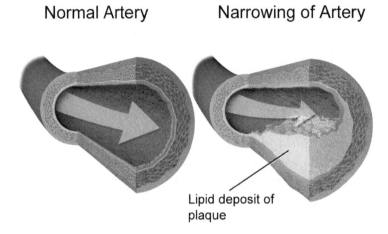

Lipid deposit of plaque

Figure 8.1: Narrowing of the coronary artery (Image by Bruce Blausen/Wikimedia).

However, newer studies show that heart attacks happen abruptly at the site of narrowing due to a sudden event, typically rupture into the plaque blocking the artery. Inflammation, similar to what you get with arthritis also plays a role. It is exceedingly rare, though not impossible, for such a complete inflammation blockage to occur at a site in the pipe that does not have plaque, so it is still necessary to control your blood cholesterol. More commonly, the artery has to be 70% narrowed or more before it is at risk from this abrupt heart-attack-causing closure.

Risk factors for CAD and heart attacks can be lumped into those you can do something about and those you can't.

8.2   CAD risk factors you can't change

Let's start with the things you can't control:

- Age

- Gender

- Family history

- Race

Typically, we consider 45 for men and 55 for women the age to begin worrying about risk of heart disease. The delayed response in women is due to a temporary hormonal benefit. However, the process occurs gradually, typically over 20 years or more, so it pays to begin early in working on those factors you can change.

Along with smoking, the strongest risk factor for heart disease is actually family history, particularly if a first-degree relative (for example, a father or sister) developed heart disease prematurely, younger than age 55. In fact, if both parents developed heart disease before age 55, your risk of having a heart attack is nearly double. You might as well take up sky diving now. The family history risk is proven in identical twin studies where one is raised with the natural parents and the other isn't. The environment (secondhand smoke, diet, and so on) is actually not very important because both twins similarly develop heart disease.[1]

Race is a minor risk factor, though. African-Americans' risk of heart disease is known to be higher due to multiple other factors (blood pressure, diet, weight, and genetics). Other races, such as Asians, have a lower risk.

Why should you care about the risk factors you can't modify? Your risk of heart disease is additive based on your risk profile. Thus, if you have the above risks, you should be even more attentive to those you *can* control.

[1] As every teenager quickly learns, blame your parents.

8.3   CAD risk factors you can change

The factors you can control:

- Cigarette smoking

- Cholesterol and other blood lipids

- Diabetes and obesity

- Hypertension and stress

8.3.1 Cigarette smoking

Cigarette smoking is the single biggest risk factor for heart disease, and even worse in women. About half of all heart attacks
in women are in those that smoke regularly or quit recently.
Male or female, smoking currently doubles your risk of getting heart disease in the next 10 years. The figure below sums
up the problem of many patients who visit the cardiologist.
Here is a woman, pregnant and smoking who is worried about
the noise from jackhammers next door to her house. It is still
common to find patients who continue to smoke yet are pre-
occupied with other less important risk factors. Don't smoke,
period.

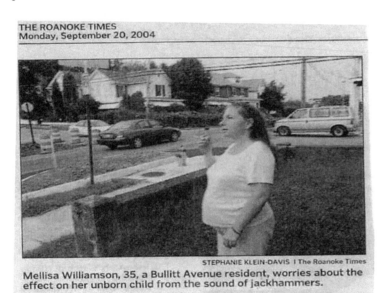

THE ROANOKE TIMES
Monday, September 20, 2004

STEPHANIE KLEIN-DAVIS | The Roanoke Times

Mellisa Williamson, 35, a Bullitt Avenue resident, worries about the
effect on her unborn child from the sound of jackhammers.

Figure 8.2: Note the
cigarette in her hand as
she worries about the sound
of jackhammers (With
permission, *The Roanoke
Times*).

8.3.2 Cholesterol and lipids

No one cared about cholesterol until the pharmaceutical industry discovered statins, those great cholesterol-lowering drugs
like Lipitor®, Zocor® and Crestor®.

The American Heart Association (AHA) got onboard with a
vengeance, particularly after some pharmaceutical donations.
Now, don't get me wrong, statins are terrific and do dramatically lower your risk of heart attack. It's just that high cholesterol itself is not a very good predictor of heart attacks (despite

the fear-mongering).

Similarly, diets focused on low fat and more carbohydrates contribute to obesity and might be counter-productive, actually increasing your risk. Also, focusing on your latest LP(a) actu-ally called "little A" lipoprotein level is far less important than just taking a statin and focusing on other reversible risk factors.

There is some truth to the cholesterol myth arguments and there is equal truth to the argument that "statins are safe and so effective they should be in the drinking water."

8.3.3   Diabetes and obesity

You might have noticed that I linked diabetes and obesity to-gether in risk-factors-you-can-change list as a single risk factor. Obesity is a risk factor for heart disease essentially only because it is associated with an increased risk of diabetes. As we get more fat cells in our body, we respond less to our naturally made insulin.

More weight equals more risk of diabetes. More diabetes equals more risk of heart disease.

Doctors used to make a big deal about Type I (insulin depen-dent) and Type II (no insulin needed) diabetes. However, this is now blurred by a flurry of strong oral diabetes medications that can be used in place of insulin. Because diabetes is such a risk factor for developing heart disease, it doesn't matter whether it is "pre-diabetes" (a term used to soften the blow that you re-ally have diabetes), insulin-dependent diabetes, or non-insulin dependent diabetes. Any kind of diabetes is bad for your heart.

While some people, particularly children, develop terrible di-abetes requiring strict insulin management their entire life, the great majority of diabetics have an acquired illness. Lose weight and the diabetes will likely disappear, often with not even that much weight loss (20 to 30 lbs). This is such an important issue that your risk of heart disease will be lowered whether you lose weight with diet, prescription medications, or bariatric surgery. "Bariatric surgery" sounds so much better than fat surgery, doesn't it? It is essentially an abdominal operation to make you feel full sooner and thus eat less. These days bariatric surgery is often done with a scope for a gastric sleeve or Lap-Band with only a small scar. Generally, bariatric surgery is reserved for those who are either 100 pounds overweight or at least 50 pounds with other weight-related reversible risk factors, like diabetes.

A word about diet drugs. Simply put, some are great, others are dangerous. We would all tolerate side effects if there was a drug that cured cancer. However, to just help with weight loss, not so much. Unfortunately, that is too often the case. Some of the new prescription meds show real promise but they are still new and diet medication side effects are often only discovered after they have been out awhile (remember Fen-Phen?).

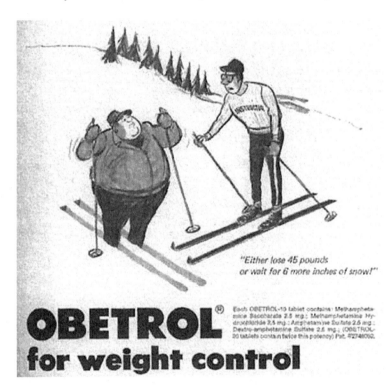

Figure 8.3: A 1970s ad for the methamphetamine diet pill Obetrol, a favorite of Andy Warhol (Photo by Rexar Pharmaceutical/Wikimedia).

Many over-the-counter supplements for diet loss are stimulants, making you feel like you slugged down a couple of espressos. As you will learn, that can carry a huge risk, especially if you have an unknown pre-existing heart condition, like an arrhythmia substrate or a low ejection fraction (EF). There is no better example than Metabolife 356, a best-selling herbal dietary supplement developed by a San Diego company. Metabolife's products were based on ephedra, a stimulant not unlike meth. In 2001, 36% of all diet pill sales in the United States were for Metabolife 356. Then, reports surfaced of heart attacks and sudden deaths. In 2004, the FDA banned its sale and the company declared bankruptcy due to a series of legal problems.

Before starting a diet drug, do your research and get a check-up, including an EKG and stress echocardiogram.

8.3.4   Hypertension and stress

By now, most everyone knows that hypertension is just a medical word for high blood pressure. It does not mean that you are "extra tense."

With myth #53 dispelled, general life stress is *not* a risk factor for hypertension or for heart disease. Hypertension and heart attacks occur in the most laid back surfer dudes you have ever seen.

Stress might indirectly affect behaviors that *do* increase heart disease risk factors, such as smoking, physical inactivity, and overeating.[2]

Science can explain some of these links between stress and modern life. The human animal developed this flight or fight response when there was a genetic advantage for the caveman. In case a saber-toothed tiger attacked, he'd be the quickest to get away. Thus, the caveman lived to breed with cave women, who looked just like Raquel Welch in *One Million Years B.C.* In this manner, the sympathetic nervous system evolved as a protective mechanism.

Have you ever had a "friend" sneak up on you and really startle you? You will get a rush of sympathetic stimulation, including the blood hormone adrenaline (also called epinephrine), causing you to become flushed, alert, and hyper-vigilant.

The general life stresses that we all recognize in today's modern world are not healthy. For example, driving on the freeway and having someone swerve into your lane isn't always a good time to have an adrenaline surge because you can overreact and cause an accident (or, even worse, get yelled at by your wife). Similarly, the whole concept of "stage fright" is the problem of excessive sympathetic stimulation at a time you would be better

[2] Americans love to blame stress for all our ills. It seems everyone has stresses to complain about, usually work related, with some inappropriately looking for a medical excuse to go on disability. By comparison, I see patients with severe heart failure and other medical problems, unable to walk 20 yards who refuse to get a disability parking placard. Guess which one I will sign the disability papers for?

served by maintaining calm. Some physicians have postulated that the common need for beta blockers, medications that block adrenaline, are a result of human's inability to adapt to modern stresses. However, it will take many generations of stress for Darwin's theory to work. It will require mating by those who handle stress without an overreaction of adrenaline.

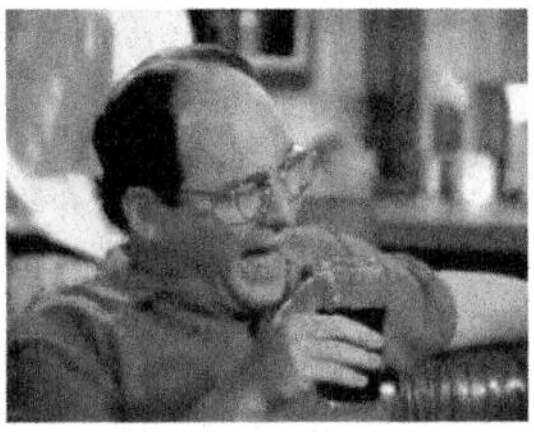

This concept of explaining mankind's evolution by the need that arises is called teleology. For example, a giraffe developed a long neck not because of stretching. The ones who were born with long necks reached the food more easily, survived, and their genes dominated the gene pool. Similarly, the human race is getting more attractive (there are noted exceptions) because beautiful people are more desired, breed more, and ugly begins to disappear or wane.

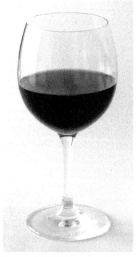

Figure 8.4: Who would you rather mate with, George Clooney or George Costanza? Men, make up your own comparison.

8.3.5 Alcohol (not a risk factor if in moderation)

I hope you noticed that alcohol is not on the list of risk factors for heart disease. Innumerable scientific studies have shown that moderate consumption of alcohol is associated with a reduction in your risk of heart disease! This is still difficult for many physicians to believe, so you might get a concerning look if you admit to a nightly drink. This attitude must stem from our Puritanical roots when doctors believed that "if it feels good, it must be bad for you."

How much is "moderate"? The standard joke is less than your doctor drinks. The science suggests that 1 to 2 drinks a day is safest; a drink defined as a beer, glass of wine, or 1 ounce of hard alcohol. Now, don't forget what your mother told you, the smartest doctor we all know, "Everything in moderation." Alcoholics have an increased risk of developing a severe heart muscle disease called alcoholic cardiomyopathy.

The data about the unique benefits of red wine is less than you might expect. I think the *French paradox* (why the French smoke, eat cheese, and don't die of heart attacks) was started by the French wine industry.

I actually attended a medical debate in France about the French paradox. The French physician talked about the benefits of the polyphenolic compounds in red wine, such as resveratrol, and how that limits the progression of plaque build-up in

Figure 8.5: The early science suggesting red wine had unique beneficial properties has not been corroborated. Probably *all* alcohol in moderation provides equal heart benefit to red wine (Photo by Andre Karwath/Wikimedia).

the arteries. At one point, a British doctor stood up and said "Do you know why the French have less heart attacks? *They can't count!* Have you ever been in a French hospital? It is full of heart attack patients."

While this anecdotal evidence isn't strong science, the real science backs up the Brit. Early research studies suggesting that red wine was the only alcohol source to decrease heart disease have not been duplicated. From a heart perspective, drinking any type of alcohol is OK in moderation. Doctor's permission.

8.4   Blood pressure

As mentioned, high blood pressure is the same as hypertension. There are many misconceptions about blood pressure but the old adage, the "silent killer," still applies. Long-standing high blood pressure causes downstream or "end" organ damage, such as thickening of the heart walls (ventricular hypertrophy), kidney failure, accelerated atherosclerosis (hardening of the arteries) of the heart, and elsewhere. About three-quarters of patients who have a stroke have a history of hypertension.

How do you know if you have high blood pressure? Check it frequently, preferably with your own blood pressure cuff at home. The trip to the doctor's office is often associated with stress (see above about the imaginary wife yelling at you in the car) both related to the travel, waiting room, and the actual visit.[3] "White coat hypertension" is a real malady, but people also use this excuse for what is real, treatable hypertension. Non-medication treatments, such as dieting, low salt intake, and even yoga sometimes work but usually for mild hypertension. Don't delay too long with these options because the effects of hypertension are cumulative. You might be damaging your end organs, which can't be a good thing.

Recent research has dispelled many of the old myths about hypertension:

- Systolic hypertension (the top number only) carries no risk.

- Mild hypertension is normal because everyone has it.

- Blood pressure medications are riskier than the problem.

[3] As you might expect, after thousands of surgeries, I have accumulated a few waiting room stories. I have spoken to the wrong family. I frequently forget the patient's name. I have also had a patient ask me to talk to his wife in one waiting room and his girlfriend in another.

None of these statements is considered true today. The most recent data does show that up to one in three adults have hypertension and it is directly associated with a greater risk of health care problems. There are many definitions of what constitutes a blood pressure-warranting treatment, but generally they are consistent blood pressure readings of 140/90 or higher. Some doctors argue for even lower values to begin treatment. Cardiologists used to manage hypertension but it is a primary care condition today because it is so prevalent and because repeated visits might be necessary to confirm proper control.

Older than 55	1 point
Ever smoked?[a]	1 point
Still smoke, after 20 years	1 more point
Family history[b]	2 points
Cholesterol ever over 225[c]	1 point
BP ever more than 150/95[c]	1 point
Diabetes or pre-diabetes[c]	1 point
Male	1 point

Table 8.1: Heart attack risk calculator.

No points	1%
1-2	5%
3-4	12%
5-8	20%
Over 8	Call the priest

Table 8.2: Estimated risk of a heart attack in the next 10 years.

a. At least 1 pack per day for 10 years, called 10 pack years to get one point.

b. Direct relative, parent, or sibling with heart attack, bypass surgery, or stent before age 55.

c. You have the risk and get a point if you ever were told you had this problem, even if it is now controlled.

The table shown is a simple approximation of your risk of heart attack based on these risk factors. My disclaimer applies here. Listen to your mother and see your doctor.

Buy an inexpensive Omron-type home blood pressure monitor and check your own blood pressure and your family's regularly. Write the numbers down and bring it to your doctor. It could save your life.

There are more than 50 medicines used to treat hypertension. Often, when there are that many medicines for a condition, none of them work very well. This generalization isn't true for hypertension; the drugs do work. Recent evidence suggests that it is actually better to take more than one medicine for hypertension because two or three medications in low dose will control it better and result in fewer side effects. The classes of common medicines for hypertension include diuretics, kidney-active drugs, like angiotension converting enzyme (ACE) inhibitors and angiotension receptor blockers (ARBs), beta blockers, calcium blockers, and others. They come in pill form and even long-acting patches.

Some people love to ask for tests to help them uncover hidden health problems. Unfortunately, that doesn't always work in their best interest. For example, healthy teenagers without risk factors don't benefit from heart screening tests because they are more likely to be falsely positive, and lead to further risky tests. If you are healthy, be skeptical of risky medical tests. However, you likely do have some risks or you wouldn't have read this far. We have already touched on getting a fasting lipid panel blood test to help determine if your cholesterol and related components are high. Other screening tests include ultrafast CT heart scans to get your calcium score. This fad is decreasing in number for the same reason. An asymptomatic patient with calcium in his heart arteries might lead to a coronary angiogram and complications for something that did not warrant treatment.

Which single number is most useful in predicting your risk of heart-related death? Cholesterol? Nope. Weight? Nope.

It is your *ejection fraction (EF)*. Our hearts pump out blood (eject it) from the major pumping chamber, the left ventricle, with each beat. A normal EF is 55 to 70%, which means that about two-thirds of the blood is ejected with each beat leaving a little behind for the next beat. Very rarely, too high of an EF can be associated with other heart and non-cardiac problems. However, a low EF is usually the problem. How low is too low? Good question. Recent data show that patients with EFs decreased to just 50% have an increased risk of heart failure. When we talk about defibrillators, you'll see that pioneering work, like the MADIT II trial, found an EF of 30% is all you need to justify protection from an implantable cardioverter defibrillator (ICD) because sudden death is very common. Thus, everyone should know their EF.

8.5   Arrhythmia risk factors

I almost forgot that this is a book about arrhythmias. Are there specific risk factors for arrhythmias? Absolutely. Of course, it depends on which arrhythmia you want to consider.

8.5.1   Sudden death risk

As I mentioned, the best predictor of your risk of a life-threatening ventricular arrhythmia is based on just one number, your EF:

- Less than 50%: See a cardiologist.

- Less than 40%: Ask to see an EP specialist; you should be on heart failure meds too.

- Less than 30%: Get an ICD evaluation now.

- Less than 25%: See a heart failure specialist too; you might need an artificial heart (LVAD).

- Less than 10%: The priest will call you.

8.5.2   Atrial fibrillation (AF) risk factors

Although there is no accepted risk factor scale for risk of developing AF, that won't stop me from making an educated guess based on my clinical experience. The goal is to realize that these risks add to your likelihood of AF.

Hypertension, BP more than 135/90	1 point
CAD or prior myocardial infarction	1 point
Heart failure diagnosis	1 point
EF less than 40%	1 point
Valvular heart disease[a]	2 points
Pericarditis in the past	1 point
Sleep apnea	1 point
Family history[b]	0 points

Table 8.3: AF risk calculator.

a. Valvular heart disease is subjective but includes an echocardiogram showing at least "moderate" (also called 2+) aortic or mitral stenosis or regurgitation. A history of rheumatic heart disease also qualifies.

b. The genetics of AF are very complex because the disease is very common. Family history is not a risk factor.

Add up your points. If you have two or more, you should be seeing a cardiologist regularly and having non-invasive screening of your heart rhythm to see if you develop AF. Remember that AF can be a silent killer too; half of patients are unaware they are in this abnormal rhythm.

8.5.3 Risk of stroke in AF

Some knucklehead came up with the terminology CHADS for a scoring system to evaluate the risk of stroke in AF.[4] CHADS actually stands for **C**ongestive heart failure, **H**ypertension, **A**ge, **D**iabetes, and **S**troke. To make matters worse, it has been modified by adding vascular heart disease and advanced age. CHA2DS2Vasc is now abbreviated, as only physicians can do, to CHADSVasc.

[4] CHADS sounds like a cute surfer dude rather than a serious scale for stroke risk.

Then, some other "me too" knucklehead recognized that gender is another risk factor. Women are more likely to get strokes probably because men die earlier from other preventable causes. Fortunately, they haven't made the CHADSVasc name any more cumbersome, adding an 'F' for female or a 'B' for black, a further stroke risk factor. If you have AF, you should know your CHADSVasc score.

CHF or EF ≤ 40%	1 point
Hypertension	1 point
Age ≥ 65	1 point
Age ≥ 75	1 more point
Diabetes	1 point
Stroke/TIA in the past	2 points
Vascular disease	1 point
Sex is female	1 point

Moderate to high risk ≥ 2

Low risk = 0-1

Table 8.4: How to calculate your CHADSVasc score (adapted from Lip and Halperin "Improving stroke risk stratification in atrial fibrillation"). See table 8.5 to calculate your risk of a stroke.

The risk of stroke in AF is also vitally important to know. While the scale we now use is applied only to people with known prior AF, some data suggest that is insignificant. If you have a high CHADSVasc score and do not yet have AF, you might still be at risk, so:

1. Get a long-term heart monitor to screen for AF.

2. Discuss the pros and cons of anticoagulation regardless of AF.

The reason this CHADSVasc scoring is important is that it reliably predicts your risk of having a stroke, a complication of AF, which is potentially preventable with blood thinners.[5] The table shown illustrates that risk is almost identical to the number of points, at least up to CHADSVasc 5, when it is even higher than 5% a year.

[5] Lip, Gregory Y.H. and Halperin, Jonathan L. "Improving stroke risk stratification in atrial fibrillation." *The American Journal of Medicine*, 123(6):484-488, June 2010.

CHADSVasc score	Patients (n = 7,329)	Adjusted stroke rate (%/year)
0		
1	422	1.3
2	1,230	2.2
3	1,730	3.2
4	1,718	4.0
5	1,159	6.7
6	679	9.8
7	294	9.6
8	82	6.7
9	14	15.2

Table 8.5: CHADSVasc score predicts annual stroke risk in AF (European Society of Cardiology. "Guidelines for the management of atrial fibrillation." *European Heart Journal*, 13(7):2369-2429, July 2010).

A good rule of thumb is that each point equals another 1% annual stroke risk (that is, 3 points = 3% annual risk of stroke). Because no one wants a stroke, what does a 1% annual risk really mean? Don't you want that risk to be zero? Unfortunately, based on a large population, 1% per year is about your baseline risk, depending on your age, even if you don't have AF. If you're younger than 65, about 0.5% a year, older than 75, about 1.2% a year. If your CHADSVasc score is really just 0 or 1, there is no data that the risks of taking a blood thinner, or even aspirin, are worth it.

What *do* you do if your CHADSVasc score is 2 or higher and thus your annual risk of stroke is 2% or higher?

That's where blood thinners come into play. Again, a good rule of thumb is to consider a blood thinner more potent than aspirin if your score is 2 or higher. Don't forget this scale is your annual risk of stroke. If you don't have one this year, the risk is the same next year and the year after. That is what pays for all those commercials about anticoagulant medicines. Unfortunately, they are followed by the lawyer commercials: "Did you bleed on an anticoagulant? Call 1-800-CHEAT-EM."[6]

8.6   Wrap

Risk factors are opportunities—opportunities to modify your personal risk of a health problem. Knowledge is power. If you know that you have an especially high risk of heart attack, perhaps because your dad had one at age 45, then that should give you extra motivation to not smoke, avoid obesity, and control your blood pressure and diabetes. Control of your risks is up to you. It might require some will power, such as to take a medicine every day, but don't you think that is worthwhile if it could prevent the problem?

I hope that you have also learned the importance of knowing how strong your heart muscle pump is, measured as EF. I wish there was as strong an ad campaign about knowing your EF as there is for knowing your cholesterol. More lives would be saved.

AF carries its own risk factor issues, primarily related to stroke risk. The research is clear about the CHADSVasc score; if yours is 2 or higher, you probably need a blood thinner.

Amazingly, motivation becomes a major issue. The real problem is that if your blood thinner prevents you from having a stroke, you'll never know it. Thus, the medicine just seems like another needless chore, yet might silently be saving your life. My mother always said, "Take your medicine and listen to your doctor." Of course, she was referring to my dad, also a physician and the one who dished out the discipline. I also remember that she said, "Just wait until your father gets home!"

[6] Did you ever wonder why they were allowed to name Apple Computers when there was already an Apple Records (the Beatles' label)? The Beatles' lawyers did too. With a straight face, Apple Computers told Apple Records that a computer would never play sounds or music. Apple Records fell for it. When the Macintosh came out, this new Apple computer had alert sounds. The very first sound was called Sosumi (So sue me, get it?). As you would expect, the Beatles didn't like that too much. Years later, they were still mad, resulting in the temporary refusal by Apple Records to allow Beatles music on iTunes.

9
Diet and over-the-counter drugs

We all want to take control of our health, and certainly heart disease is one major problem we would love to prevent. Unfortunately, there is an incredible amount of nonsense out there about alternative opportunities, many foisted on an unsophisticated public who believe what they read. Some of this is amplified by "traditional" medicine experts who might have a different agenda than your health.

Before we address some of the benefits of diets and over-the-counter drugs, let's look at some of these myths.

9.1 Myths about heart disease and arrhythmia

Here are five myths about heart disease that can help you when considering diet and medicines:

1. Diet can substantially reduce your chance of getting heart disease.

2. Avoiding stimulants will prevent you from getting an arrhythmia.

3. CoQ10 and Omega-3 fish oil are proven to be helpful for your heart.

4. The FDA can't be trusted.

5. Prescription medications are safer than over-the-counter drugs.

9.1.1   Myth 1: Diet can substantially reduce your chance of getting heart disease

We discussed the impact of diet on standard coronary disease in the previous chapter. The focus on one food group, whether that is avoiding fat or avoiding carbohydrates is much less important than you might think. Long-term, a low-fat diet can reduce your bad cholesterol (LDL), but short-term, it has no benefit. Lowering your bad cholesterol with a low-fat diet sounds good, but does this prevent heart disease? Not really. The USDA food guide pyramid has been discarded because the concept of a low-fat diet has not reduced heart disease in populations as large as 50,000 studied (for example, the Women's Health Initiative Dietary Modification Trial). Now, don't run out and eat a slab of bacon, but relax about low fat.

The Atkins diet craze of low carbohydrates was lambasted by cardiologists because less carbs resulted in more fat and protein intake. Don't forget that there are only three types of foods that provide any calories: carbohydrates, protein, and fats, that's it. This low-carb-oriented diet can reduce heart disease primarily due to the associated weight loss. This diet was popular because it generates quick water loss, which motivates those involved to continue. However, it has never been shown to be that helpful.

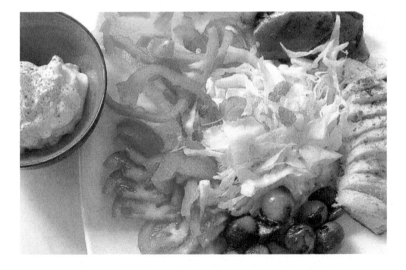

Figure 9.1: A typical Atkins diet meal (Photo by Amontillado/Wikimedia).

America is getting fatter. There is such a temptation to try the next fad diet that the hucksters are everywhere. They prey on our desire for a simple solution to weight loss and heart health. Just recently, one such fad was the pH Miracle, an alkaline diet touted as "The New Biology." Popular products included Cardio Health, just $25 for a 7-day supply, advertised with careful wording "believed to help relieve heart failure." The proponent, Robert Young, PhD, was accused of defrauding patients at his $2,000-a-day retreat where he administered pH-balancing diet therapy (even giving intravenous baking soda). In February 2016, Mr. Young was convicted of practicing medicine without a license. By the way, "Doctor" Young received his PhD from a non-accredited defunct correspondence school in Alabama. He is now in jail. Buyer beware.

So, what can you do? While there is no magic diet restriction or additive that will prevent heart disease, anything that will reduce obesity and diabetes is helpful. One option is to try the "Mama Told Me" diet. Eat everything in moderation, reducing overall calories. Another option pick a reasonably safe fad diet, lose weight, and keep it off, knowing that the goal of weight loss is its associated reduction in Type II diabetes. If cutting out gluten makes you eat less, that helps, though it might have nothing to do with the gluten avoidance itself. That is about all you can do.

9.1.2 Myth 2: Avoiding stimulants will prevent you from getting an arrhythmia

The diet advice related to arrhythmias generally focuses on stimulant intake. Stimulants come in numerous forms but are all related to adrenaline, also called epinephrine, the body's natural fight-or-flight hormone.

These stimulants include prescription drugs, such as Ritalin, used to treat ADHD, which apparently is as common as coffee in college libraries. Illegal stimulants include cocaine, ecstasy (also called MDMA), and others. The most famous legal stimulant is caffeine, the drug that created a Fortune 200 company, Starbucks.[1] Of course, caffeine isn't as awful as ecstasy, but don't forget it is a stimulant. Other common legal stimulants include pseudoephedrine (Sudafed®), which these

[1] Starbucks is not alone but is an amazing story: 20 straight years of 5% growth or more, nearly 25,000 stores in 66 countries all based around a culture of caffeine enjoyment.

days you must purchase from behind the counter at most phar-
macies because it is used to make illegal methamphetamine
(crystal meth). Decongestants with phenylpropanolamine (PPA)
are also stimulants, found in common cough and cold over-
the-counter medications like some versions of Robitussin®,
Triaminic®, and so on. Recently, many PPA products have been
pulled because of a risk of brain bleeding and stroke.

Now all these stimulants aren't equivalent, but any of them
can be bad for you if you have arrhythmias as well as other
heart problems, like hypertension or coronary heart disease.
With arrhythmias, the problem is two-fold. Stimulants increase
the number of premature beats from the upper or lower chambers, called SVEs or PVCs.[2] While we all have some of these
extra beats, the stimulant meds cause more. These beats contribute to more serious arrhythmias in two ways:

- **Increased episodes of heart racing if you have a pre-
  existing substrate.** Many people are unaware that they
  might have an abnormality of two pathways inside their
  heart, instead of the usual one. More extra beats results in
  more chances the wires will get crossed and cause arrhythmias, such as common supraventricular tachycardias (SVTs)
  like AV node reentrant tachycardia or atrial flutter.

- **Increased rate or frequency of non-substrate arrhythmias.**
  Whether atrial fibrillation (AF), inappropriate sinus tachycardia, or other fast heart rhythms, stimulants make them go
  even faster. Obviously, a heart rate of 200 is worse than 150.

Regardless, strict avoidance of stimulants will never completely prevent arrhythmias, though they might make them so
infrequent it becomes tolerable. Switch to decaf.

9.1.3   Myth 3: CoQ10 and Omega-3 fish oil are proven helpful for your heart

Coenzyme Q10, CoQ10, is commonly touted as a dietary supplement to cure what ails you—from high blood pressure to
depressed immune function to high cholesterol to dementia to
cancer to low sperm count (not necessarily a bad thing anyway). It is a natural enzyme involved in creating the power
source in our bodies, adenosine triphosphate (ATP). But does

[2] Remember the first rule of med school? SVEs stands for supraventricular ectopics and PVCs stands for premature ventricular contractions. Medical words must be longer than normal words.

that mean that taking it as a dietary supplement works? In short, no. In exhaustive reviews of the available science, both the American Heart Association (AHA) and the National Institutes of Health (NIH) have found no believable scientific evidence that CoQ10 helps. However, in reasonable doses (3 grams a day or less), it probably is not harmful; now isn't that a rousing endorsement?

At first blush, fish oils sounded like a good idea. It is common knowledge that cultures that eat a lot of fresh fish (Japanese, Inuits) have a much lower incidence of heart disease. Unfortunately, these advantages are not bestowed on those who eat fried fish. Why eat an oily fish when you can take a pill? Hence the popularity of marine omega-3 fatty acid fish oil supplements.

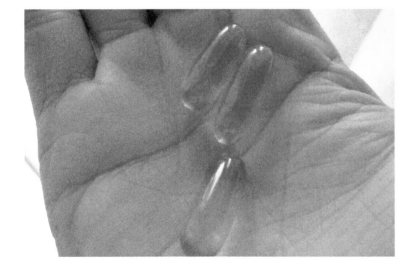

Figure 9.2: Fish oil capsules (Adapted from Stephen Cummings/Flickr).

There actually is a lot of science on omega-3 fish oil supplements. Most of the studies were done on high-risk patients who had known high cholesterol and/or hypertension and were also on prescription medicines. A summary (called a meta-analysis) of 14 randomized (patients didn't know if they were taking placebo or fish oil) studies involving thousands of patients concluded that "omega-3 fish oil supplements do not prevent cardiovascular disease." Another myth busted. There might be a minor role in selected patients who have a relatively rare isolated high triglyceride problem. In addition, there remains a likely benefit of eating fresh fish in your diet; the AHA recommends at least twice a week.

Especially in California, it is extremely common to find people who trust what they read on the label in the vitamin store and are taking five or 10 "supplements" that they swear by. These over-the-counter medications do not have to prove their value. Hiding behind First Amendment freedom of speech, over-the-counter supplement makers can claim whatever they want. You must be proactive about your own health and question whatever you read.[3]

[3] With the exception of this book, of course.

9.1.4 Myth 4: The FDA can't be trusted

The U.S. government established the Food and Drug Administration in 1906 to regulate misbranded food and drugs. Since then, the FDA has evolved into a huge government bureaucracy (stop me if you have heard this before) annually spending more than $5 billion in tax dollars as well as getting additional revenue from drug and device companies who want their products to be reviewed. Besides the bloated budget, there have been many criticisms of the FDA. These include *over-regulation* that delays worthwhile drug approval (because an FDA bureaucrat has never been promoted for approving a drug). On the contrary, almost daily, someone at the FDA points to the FDA's efficiency in preventing Thalidomide, the anti-nausea pregnancy drug, from approval in the United States. Thalidomide was later found to cause horrible birth defects (babies born with severely deformed limbs). Unfortunately, the real story was that the FDA delayed Thalidomide only because it was stuck on some employee's desk, not because of concern about its dangers. It has been suggested that the inordinate delays at the FDA have caused more deaths than lives saved.

The FDA has also been criticized for *under-regulation*, approving unsafe products like Vioxx and some food additives. It's really a damned if you do, damned if you don't scenario. Unfortunately, the First Amendment interpretation has recently resulted in the FDA being restricted in what they are willing to prevent drug and device companies from saying in advertisements. Even prescription products can now make unverified claims.

After all this criticism, you must be wondering how is it a myth that "the FDA can't be trusted?" I view the FDA like Winston Churchill viewed democracy:

> Democracy is the worst form of government, except for all the others.

Despite its problems, the FDA is the best regulatory agency in the world reviewing the safety of food, drugs, and devices. They require rigorous testing before they will approve a prescription medicine, a job that has saved countless American lives. An FDA approval means that a prescription medicine has undergone many years of study in animals and then people to prove that is is safe and effective. The exceptions make big news, but the FDA does a tremendous job most of the time.

9.1.5   Myth 5: Prescription medications are safer than over-the-counter drugs

Taken as a group, prescription medications do pose more risks than over-the-counter drugs. That is because many of the over-the-counter drugs are placebos, formulations with no active ingredients, or in extremely low doses. They don't work but they usually don't hurt either (if you don't count that hurt to your wallet). As part of their safety mandate, all prescription meds have a long list of side effects easily accessible to the consumer now with access to the Internet. This list often causes more confusion than help. Can you blame an uninformed citizen who chooses to not take a prescribed medicine after reading it might cause you to grow a second head? No wonder people turn to the unregulated supplement market, which has no such mandate to list side effects or proof that it works. However, remember that mom also said, "Don't believe everything you read."

The FDA approaches over-the-counter dietary supplements (they won't even call them medicines) "under a different set of regulations than those covering 'conventional' foods and drug products." Essentially, they just regulate whether the supplements are "adulterated or misbranded." All they can say is that you can't sell motor oil and call it fish oil. But, they have intentionally avoided evaluating the efficacy of these supplements.

Much of the time, you don't know if they do what they claim. However, a little common sense applies. If you invented a supplement that you were convinced really saved lives, wouldn't you want to sponsor serious research and submit it for FDA approval to validate your claims?

As an informed patient, you should consider the risk-reward with any medication prescribed, or for that matter, any invasive procedure or surgery recommended.[4] Ask your physician and do your own research on the risk of no treatment in addition to the risk of the medication or surgery. I recently had a patient who had a 1 in 100 serious ablation complication, called tamponade where her blood pressure dropped because blood was squeezing the outside of the heart from a little hole that the catheter caused. Fortunately, it was promptly recognized and treated. Instead of going home that day, she awakened in the ICU with a drainage catheter in the sack around her heart. She quickly healed and was discharged the next day without long-term injury. She concluded, "Even if someone had told me I would have had this complication, I would have still proceeded. I am so delighted my PVCs and VT have been cured. Thank you, doc." Even after the rare complication, she understood that the risk-reward was in her favor. In electrophysiology (EP), thanks are rare but always welcome.

9.2   Other quackery

Most of the claims written on dietary supplements in health food stores are not confirmed. Similarly, others are preying on your interest in maintaining good health. One other area you might not be so aware of is lab testing. The FDA has recently recognized that lab testing is the "Wild West" of medicine, as controversial journalist Tom Burton of *The Wall Street Journal* put it.[5] Of course, most routine lab work is regulated and accurate. However, there is big money in doing unusual tests, often developed by the labs themselves. Amazingly, the Mayo Clinic has leveraged its name into a huge business of doing a lot of these lab tests of uncertain benefit, to the tune of $600 million a year.

Unproven but marketed blood tests that the FDA and others have questioned include:

[4] People often struggle with relative risk. You can consider this like cost-benefit or risk-reward theory. Seat belts are a good example. My sweet mother-in-law, Grandma Marge, won't wear her seat belt because she has read about people who have had chest injuries from being restrained. There is also the mythical story of the car accident victim who was saved by being thrown through the windshield avoiding injuries in the vehicle. Developed 50 years ago by Volvo, the seat belt has been described as "the most effective safety device ever invented," clearly having saved more than 1 million lives. I haven't heard of 1 million people being safely thrown out the windshield from their crashed car.

[5] Burton, Thomas M. "Is Lab Testing the 'Wild West' of Medicine?" *The Wall Street Journal*, December 2015.

- Heart screening, like homocysteine, vitamin D, and the KIF6 gene test

- Some ovarian cancer screening blood tests

- Colon cancer screening with Septin 9 (rejected by FDA but marketed anyway)

- Lyme disease blood screening

- Autism (the Maternal-Antibody-Related autism or MAR test)

- Routine prostate-specific antigen testing in men with no symptoms of prostate problems

Of course, many screening lab tests have value, particularly when used on the right risk group. Genetic testing in patients with congenital conditions like Long QT syndrome and a risk of sudden death can help determine the risk in family members, guiding treatment.

While I am generally opposed to government overregulation, I do believe that the public is being scammed into paying for unnecessary lab tests with no proven value. In 2013, the FDA did step in and required 23andMe to stop selling its popular genetic screening test because they were marketing benefits far beyond its proven value. Recently, however, these genetic screening tests are back on the market with more restrictive benefit claims. The FDA has been reluctant to criticize companies with obviously false medical marketing claims stating that restricting ads impinges on the companies' right of free speech. To me, this is like shouting "Fire!" in a crowded theater, not protected free speech. In my opinion, some medical marketing claims should be illegal because the public can be avoidably harmed.

The FDA has a responsibility to protect the unknowing public.

9.3   Snake oil salesmen like Dr. Oz

We all want an easy way to get healthy because the hard way of losing weight and exercising is no fun at all, and it doesn't even work a lot of the time people try it. This is a perfect setup for con artists, referred to as snake oil salesmen, because snake

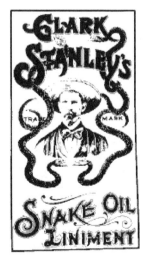

Figure 9.3: Clark Stanley's Snake Oil liniment.

oil used to be a "cure all" product you could buy. In 1917, the U.S. government tested Stanley's Snake Oil and found that it contained mineral oil, 1% fatty oil, red pepper, turpentine, and camphor but did not contain any actual snake oil. The government sued Clark Stanley, the "Rattlesnake King," and subsequently snake oil became a term for false cures.

Today, snake oils are everywhere from TV commercials about a "100% digital" device that cures your arthritis to nearly every product in the "health" food store to Dr. Oz.

The last one drives me crazy. Oz is actually Dr. Mehmet Cengiz Öz, son of Turkish immigrants, who must have been really smart when he was young because he attended Harvard for his BA and MD and Penn's Wharton School of Business for his MBA degree. He went on to become a skilled heart surgeon at Columbia University in New York where he conducted research on normal things, like minimally invasive cardiac surgery.

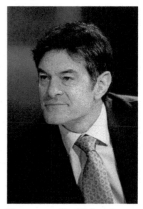

Figure 9.4: Dr. Mehmet Oz in 2012 (Photo by the World Economic Forum/Wikimedia).

At some point, he must have bumped his head really hard. In truth, I suspect the economics of practicing medicine today got the best of him. "All those years, long hours, and for what? An income that won't allow me to afford a home in Manhattan?" So Oz went the alternative route and to the extreme. Starting with Oprah, and then on his own, he learned that if he promoted items like resveratrol to prevent aging, people gobbled it up, not only tuning in but indirectly paying him a fortune in the process.

Oz has been outed by responsible journalists and scientists, though it is too little too late. Colleagues at Columbia got fed up and wrote the Dean:

> Oz ... is guilty of either outrageous conflicts of interest or flawed judgments.

They deemed "his presence on the faculty of a prestigious medical institution unacceptable." An article in the *British Medical Journal* found that 54% of his recommendations had no scientific backing or rationale, 15% directly against scientific evidence.[6] *Popular Science* and *The New Yorker* have published articles criticizing Oz for "doing more harm than good."

Dr. Oz's Harvard and Wharton education was not wasted; he just uses it now to skirt the law. As Oz laughs all the way to the bank, innocent viewers avoid seeing their doctors in hopes that

[6] Korownyk, Christina et al. "Televised medical talk shows—what they recommend and the evidence to support their recommendations." 2014. http://www.bmj.com/content/349/bmj.g7346.

his latest "cure" (avoid apple juice because it contains arsenic, use Reiki energy therapy to find your chi, drink green coffee bean extract to lose weight, and so on) will save them.

How does Oz get away with it? He cleverly quotes others when endorsing a product as a recent Reddit article "Why is Dr. Oz allowed?" described:[7]

> Oz will state, "What options are there for people with itchy feet? Well, a recent study found that 57% of people who eat dryer lint say their feet do not itch."

By the way, except for the dryer lint, all these are real Oz recommendations. Just wait until he gets ahold of that one, there will be a sudden shortage of dryer lint saved by a new Oz endorsed product "Lint 4 You."

[7] DanaNotDonna. "Why are shows like Dr. Oz allowed to give out health advice that isn't scientifically supported?" 2015. https://www.reddit.com/r/explainlikeimfive/comments/3u1gjr/eli5_why_are_shows_like_droz_allowed_to_give_out/.

9.4   Health foods

Did you know that you cannot label foods like salmon, avocado, or nuts as "healthy?" It has to be a processed food to get that label. Of course, there are FDA standards so that not all processed foods can market that they are healthy, but the FDA standards are questionable. My suggestion is to ignore the healthy label altogether when deciding on foods.

Similarly, labels like "fat-free" or "all natural" might be on foods that are not healthy at all. As long as you don't add colors or artificial flavors you can call it all natural. It is fine to inject them with sodium, high fructose corn syrup, and other "natural" substances. Also, when shopping for healthy bread, don't get fooled by the term "multigrain," which can include oatmeal, brown rice, and popcorn. Some, even have caramel color added to make them look darker and thus, presumably healthier. Look for terms like whole grain or 100% whole wheat, which are better choices.

The public is learning the risks of "natural" foods with the outbreak of E. coli food-borne illnesses at Chipotle and other restaurants. One reason for Chipotle's success with their high-calorie burrito restaurants is their marketing that they are better because they use unprocessed "fresh" or raw ingredients. They tout: "Great ingredients make great-tasting food." No argument there.

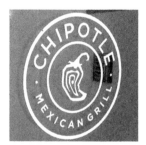

Figure 9.5: The Chipotle logo at a Chipotle in West Hartford, CT (Modified from Mike Mozart/Flickr).

However, they go on to mention that their great ingredients are "responsibly raised meats, organic agriculture, pasture-raised dairy, cooked only with non-GMO ingredients." I already feel better eating that 1,000-calorie burrito because it is fresh and natural. Unfortunately, such practices translate into greater risk of food-borne illness. There is nothing to protect you from the potentially unsanitary harvesting of such ingredients by migrant workers and those involved in the food handling chain. Is "fresher" food worth the risk? The industrialized food processing that we have learned to despise might actually make our food safer.

Many scientists have suggested that irradiating these fresh ingredients is a great solution because this kills most bacteria, fungi, insects, and molds, yet diminishes the need for processed ingredients. Radiation does not reduce nutrients in the food and causes no long-term health risks (no, it doesn't make food radioactive). Two organizations that are rarely on the same page, the FDA and *Mother Jones* (a left-leaning magazine) have encouraged irradiation of foods. We don't think twice about consuming pasteurized milk or pressure-canned foods, processes that were adopted to kill bacteria. Perhaps someday, irradiation of fresh food will be considered an equally safe and routine practice.

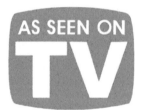

Figure 9.6: A typical "As seen on TV" sticker used to advertise many products (Modified from Radiant chains/Wikimedia).

Now, you might have a hard time believing that the latest gospel about diet and over-the-counter medications might *not* be true. The food industry and snake oil salesmen have saturated the airwaves with health foods, so it must be true because you saw it on TV. Not so fast. All I ask is that you have a little healthy skepticism and read from reliable sources, not someone who stands to gain from your gullibility. As Mark Twain said, "It ain't what you don't know that gets you into trouble. It's what you know for sure that just ain't so."

The ancient Greek philosopher Aristotle first said, "moderation in all things."[8]

[8] A recently uncovered tweet from Aristotle's mother reads: "Now Ari, please change that to everything in moderation, except bacon."

9.5   Wrap

We have reviewed a lot of myths, which is code for misinformation (which can be code for lies), about diet and over-the-counter medicines that prevent heart disease. That doesn't

mean that every non-prescription option is bad. It is just a reminder to always question your source and investigate the
science behind claims before jumping in.

What are some diet and exercise things you can do to dimin-
ish your risk or frequency of arrhythmias?

- If there is a "trigger"—whether exercise, caffeine, or something else—stop it! (Medical school rule number four: If it
  hurts when you do that, don't do that.)

- If you have a known arrhythmia, avoid stimulants from
  caffeine to diet drugs to illegal stimulants.

- Enjoy everything in moderation (including diet, exercise,
  sodium, and alcohol).[9]

- Avoid quackery and unproven cures.

- Minimize your coronary artery disease (CAD) risk factors.
  - Keep your weight down with any diet that works for you.
  - Don't ever smoke cigarettes.
  - Make sure your blood pressure is normal.
  - Get a lipid panel blood test.

- Get an echocardiogram or other test to determine your ejection fraction (EF)

- Learn more about your own health by reading up (like you
  are doing!).

[9] A couple of years ago, a friend was in a Chinese restaurant and found only a red-topped soy sauce bottle on his table. He asked the proprietor for the green-lid, lower-in-sodium type. In a heavy accent, the Asian proprietor said, "All same." My friend again explained that no, he preferred the low sodium green-lid type. This went on for a while until, exasperated, the restaurant owner finally showed him a large plastic container of soy sauce kept in the back, "All same, all same."

10
Finding the right doctor

So, you need a good doctor? Let's start with two simple questions:

1. Does your insurance plan limit who you can see?

2. Do you have a trusted primary care doctor?

10.1 *Does your insurance plan limit who you can see?*

Many insurance plans—whether HMOs, PPOs, or a variant—have in-plan and out-of-plan physicians. If you go to an out-of-plan doctor, there's an extra charge for your visit, sometimes quite substantial. Most of the time, you can find an excellent doctor who has contracted with your plan. Get the list and start your research. If you can't find who you need, call and complain. You will find this is an invaluable tool in today's complex health insurance market. Insurance companies live in fear of complaints to the state insurance commission, so you can sometimes encourage them to do what is right by a gentle reminder of your power.

One of the most useful pieces of information for dealing with insurance companies in any capacity is: *be your own advocate*. The vocal patient, the "squeaky wheel," will often get an approval when the quiet, nice guy will get denied.

10.2 *Do you have a trusted primary care doctor?*

These days, the answer is frequently no. Obviously, if you have one, ask your doctors about your physician specialist needs.

Not only are primary care providers (PCPs) a great source, it is likely the referral will result in good communication with your PCP. By the way, PCP is now the term most commonly used for internists, family physicians, including office-based Ob/Gyn doctors, pediatricians and even some office-based cardiologists.

The finances of practicing medicine today are increasingly challenging. PCPs often have to decide between joining a medical group that limits their patient contact time (some see as many as 12 patients an hour) or doing *concierge medicine*. Concierge medicine is essentially confirmation that our current health system, with or without the Affordable Care Act (ACA, also commonly known as ObamaCare), has failed. Some like to paint it as a return to the age when doctors made house calls and saw patients directly. You decide. Essentially, these doctors have restricted their practice, from up to 3,000 patients to less than 500 who now receive more "focused" care. For a substantial extra fee, on top of your insurance payment, you can now have access to what often is a reliably attentive physician.

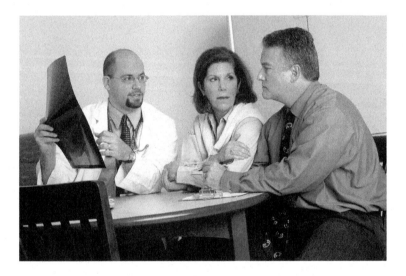

Figure 10.1: Wouldn't it be great if house calls were for everyone? (Photo by Rhoda Baer/National Cancer Institute).

These charges vary depending on location and how much access you want. In my area, the annual charges are about:

- Basic concierge access, including personal calls and improved access, $1,000/year

- Advanced access, including the doctor's cell phone and a

free annual exam, $2,500 to $5,000/year

There is even a new trend for concierge cardiology. I know one practice that gives a free AliveCor Kardia™ heart monitor along with e-mail access to the doctor to interpret rhythms for all who sign up for the $5,000 advanced care.

Unfortunately, the advent of concierge medicine leaves those who cannot afford it even less chance to see a primary care physician. If a PCP drops his patient load from 3,000 to focus on 500 who pay extra, what happens to the other 2,500?

In any other business, this would be a market-driven problem that could be fixed—if only market forces would work like that in medicine.

10.2.1   Evaluating a physician

These days, patients rarely see a new doctor without checking the doctor out online. Unfortunately, the first page of search engines are polluted with websites that don't help, unless you want to pay a fee. I would suggest caution here, ignore the national services (I can't mention any by name for obvious reasons) and get some local information. Try to find information from the doctor's own website or the doctor's hospital's site. You should be able to find a photo, credentials, and some practice information for free, though it might be on the second or third page of your search.

You'd think that a label of "Top Doctor" would tell you that you will be seeing, well, a top doctor. Not so fast, my friend. In general, the Top Doctor awards are either driven by magazines looking to sell issues or can simply be purchased from a mill. The magazines that get their rankings by polling physicians are often skewed towards doctors in large groups (for example, the Kaiser doctors will vote for other Kaiser doctors) and by the selfish thought, "If I can't vote for myself, who do I really want on the list?"

Like many doctors, in my exam room where new patients wait, I have diplomas and other items on the wall. This ranges from cherished degrees to board certifications to photos. The ones that most patients are impressed with are the Top Doctor plaques.

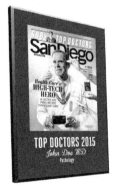

Figure 10.2: Many large city magazines have a Top Doctors issue, often a big seller (With permission, *San Diego Magazine*).

10.2.2 Board certification

You would think that a useful credential for your new doctor is board certification, but surprisingly, not always. The American Board of Internal Medicine (ABIM) regulates internal medicine physicians, cardiologists, and other medical subspecialists, such as kidney and cancer doctors. Unfortunately, they recognized that board certification is a potential profit center.

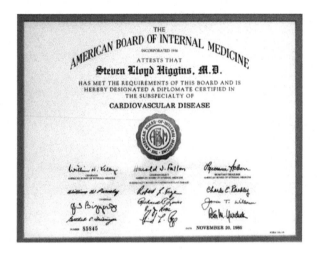

Figure 10.3: A board certificate from the ABIM, subspecialty of Cardiovascular Medicine.

At this point, the ABIM devised a 10-year mandatory renewal, ongoing annual tests on topics usually not related to patient care, expensive courses they provide to help pass the tests, and other busy work. Because no doctor wants to be considered to be against education and testing, the ABIM almost got away with it. However, the proverbial fecal material hit the fan when it was reported that ABIM executives were receiving annual salaries of $500,000 to $1,000,000, chauffeured BMWs, and personal condos paid for by physician exam fees. By the way, these doctors certifying the rest of us don't even practice medicine anymore. As a result, alternative board certification, such as the National Board of Physicians and Surgeons, have been developed by respected physicians, including my colleague, Paul Teirstein. Other excellent physicians have chosen to not renew their original board certification altogether, so that lack of board certification no longer means a physician is not competent or well trained.

With this problem, how do you assess board certification related to your new doctor? It is imperative that your physician
passes the first level of board certification after completing residency or fellowship training. This milestone guarantees that the
person has completed an approved residency, absorbed what
was needed, and is a true specialist. This initial board certification prevents you from seeing someone who just declares him-
or herself an expert in a discipline ("Free brain surgery from a
specialist!").

Being awarded the title of Fellow does mean that you completed specialized training and passed your medical board
exam. However, many physicians who are strapped for cash,
also stop paying the annual $2,000 renewal fees and stop using
the Fellow designation. Of course, that doesn't mean they are
any less talented. In my case, I am triple-boarded in internal
medicine, cardiology, and cardiac electrophysiology. However, I
no longer pay to maintain the designation FACP (Fellow of the
American College of Physicians, the internal medicine certification) or FACC (Fellow the American College of Cardiology).
I do pay the annual fee to maintain my FHRS designation, Fellow the Heart Rhythm Society, because they are good people
and I need at least one "F" after my name.

10.2.3   *Other tools to evaluate a new physician*

Do you want to know how we picked an OB doctor to deliver
our children? Although I was friends with many obstetricians, I
went to the Labor and Delivery floor and asked the experienced
nurses. These frontline workers see the doctors in action. They
honestly told me who they trusted most, an invaluable recommendation. For choosing a physician or many other health care
decisions, ask a nurse in the know.

State licensing is also a valuable resource. Most states must
publicly disclose if a physician has had sanctions leveled
against them. However, this is often not disclosed until a
lengthy review process has been completed. Some unprofes-
sional doctors never get sanctioned by their state board and,
even worse, some who aren't bad, do.

Hospital privileging is a valuable tool in judging a physician's competence. The Joint Commission: Accreditation,

Health Care, Certification previously called JCAHO (and still called "Jay-Ko" for some reason) is an independent group that scrutinizes hospital policies as well as individual physician privileges. One valuable resource is to pick a doctor who works at a Joint Commission-approved hospital.

For a procedural physician, select someone who has vast experience in both the routine and complicated procedure or surgery. Even a routine case can become a challenge that is best overcome with experience. This type of expertise only comes with *volume* of cases performed. In medicine, one highly reliable correlate of quality is simply the number of procedures the physician has performed as well as the hospital. It is no accident that the *U.S. News & World Report* list of best heart programs are also the largest programs in the country. Some might think that volume could mean a program does unnecessary procedures or is a "mill" cranking large volumes in and out for profit. Fortunately, in today's world of high scrutiny, this is rarely, if ever, the case. Don't be afraid to ask your doctor, "How many of these have you done?"[1]

A perfect example of why experience matters happened to me recently when I did a nervous young woman's "routine" ablation for supraventricular techycardia (SVT). After inserting the catheters, I discovered she had two completely unrelated serious arrhythmias, one a concealed type of Wolff-Parkinson-White syndrome (WPW)—that extra pathway some people are born with). To fix this, it required that I carefully place a needle and catheter across her heart's atrial septum to map and eliminate the extra pathway. She had a great outcome but only because the physician and hospital had vast experience in the routine and not-so-routine cases. You never want your doctor to tell your family in the waiting room "Well, I've never seen that before."

A teaching hospital provides additional challenges when evaluating a new physician. Many of the best hospitals in the world are associated with medical schools and residency programs. Doctors-in-training at these hospitals learn by doing work under supervision, whether they are interns, residents, or advanced fellows. While there is more supervision than when I trained, the "see one, do one, teach one" adage still can apply in some situations. Today, not only do you want to query the

[1] When I get this question, before answering truthfully, I can't help but tell the anxious new patient, "Well, this will be my second one but the first one should pull through ..." It always gets a laugh, albeit a nervous one.

attending doctor on his or her personal volume, but you also want to ask who actually performs the procedure. You must be an advocate for your own best care. Not to be repetitious, but did I mention that you must be an advocate for your own best care?[2]

10.2.4   *Allied health practitioners*

It is uncommon to get medical care now without running across a *physician extender*, most commonly a nurse practitioner (NP) or physician assistant (PA). I don't really like the "extenders" terminology, preferring Allied Health Practitioners or AHPs. Depending on local laws, NPs can practice medicine independently, though they must function under a physician's supervision. They can prescribe medications and often practice independently under protocols that describe their scope of practice. Thus, a cardiac EP NP can't give you Botox, nor can a dermatology NP check your defibrillator. PAs in most jurisdictions need more supervision than an NP (notes have to be co-signed daily, for example). PAs more commonly work as hospital-based surgical assistants than NPs do, but there are many exceptions.

Medicine has become so specialized that many physicians no longer are comfortable practicing outside their area of expertise. In EP, which is a sub-sub-specialty (Specialty is internal medicine, subspecialty is cardiology, thus electrophysiology really is a sub-sub).[3] NPs and PAs often do on-the-job training in one particular specialized area, such as just office practice of cardiac EP. They often become more competent than most physicians in this one area because that is all they do. In addition, my office NPs have more time (and compassion) than I do, so you are better off seeing them anyway.

I actually prefer working with NPs or PAs more than I do with residents or fellows. The physicians-in-training are often less willing to follow instructions and just after you get them trained, they move on to another rotation. However, the AHPs are often very loyal and knowledgeable in their specific area of practice. They learn how to do their work from their physician partner, so the practice routine is more consistent.

I couldn't work without these AHPs. I respect their opinion

[2] Getting the old gray-haired professor isn't always the best. I remember hearing a horrifying story from Dallas Parkland Hospital, the site where John F. Kennedy was taken after his assassination. A STAT page was placed overhead for the dean of the medical school to immediately come to the emergency room. Knowledgeable physicians in the hospital, unaware of the circumstances, quickly figured out that President Kennedy must be there and also that he would not survive. If the terrific ER and trauma staff at Parkland couldn't save him, certainly the dean wasn't going to. This overhead page is another version of "It's time to call the priest."

[3] Remember that line that I have learned more and more about less and less until now I know everything about nothing?

and clinical expertise. When you go to the office as a patient, you might likely be seeing an AHP rather than the MD unless this is a first visit or a unique situation. Please treat them with the same respect (or lack thereof) you would extend to the physician and take advantage of their experience.

10.2.5   Bedside manner

We all want our doctor to look like George Clooney and act like Marcus Welby (or Dr. House if you are younger). Of course, if your medical problem is primarily an office-based issue, like you need a good PCPs, it is important to select a physician who has good bedside manner. You want your doctor to listen to you, treat you like an individual, and take the time to explain the issues.

However, for a procedure or surgery, bedside manner is far less important than procedural experience and success rates. In fact, sometimes, it seems like the more gruff and hurried a high-volume doctor might be, the better the doctor's skills. The doctor who does three or more complex cases a day is often in a hurry, but the doctor has two attributes you must respect: procedural volume, which usually equates with best results, and the fact that others must trust this doctor or they wouldn't be so busy. This might be the reason why your doctor is abrupt.[4]

[4] As Henny Youngman explained, "A man goes to a psychiatrist. 'Nobody listens to me!' The doctor says, 'Next!' "

10.3   Choosing a health plan

Today, we don't choose doctors, we choose health plans. Most employers offer a cafeteria-style approach to choosing your insurance, usually with a maximum reimbursement that isn't enough to cover what you need. You can choose the filet mignon, but you must pay extra. When it comes to choosing health insurance, there are three major factors.[5]

10.3.1   Is my doctor included?

Obviously, if you have a doctor you love, it is important to make sure this doctor is on the plan. Call the office to ask if the plan you select is one that's accepted. Some plans are easier to work with than others in terms of pre-authorizations, ease of

[5] The 7-year-old girl told her mom, "A boy in my class asked me to play doctor." The mother nervously sighed, "Oh, dear. What happened, honey?" "Nothing, he made me wait 45 minutes and then billed my insurance for the extra time."

payment, hours on hold, and so on. Many doctors sign up for plans that might reimburse poorly just to provide care to special patients or to provide a service to their referring physicians (for example, MediCal, Medicaid).

For my practice, MediCal is actually a money loser; I pay more for my overhead than I am reimbursed from MediCal. It is my version of giving back to the community, though unlike lawyers, this type of pro bono (Latin for lawyers get to deduct it but the rest of us don't) work is not deductible.

10.3.2   Am I likely to get sick in the next year?

No one has a crystal ball about this but a personal experience is a great example. Because my wife and I are generally healthy, I choose plans with a high deductible. Amazingly, the difference between a $2,000 deductible and a $5,000 deductible plan might actually be more than $3,000 in payments during a year. With the $2,000 plan, when you get sick, your out-of-pocket cost won't be as high. However, your take-home pay will be a lot less. If you get by without using the full deductible amount you get to keep the rest. For those who are healthy, it is generally better to choose a high-deductible plan.

Recently, I took my own advice even knowing my wife's knee had been acting up lately. You guessed it, after various treatments, she underwent a knee replacement last year. Brilliantly, I had selected a $10,000 deductible plan to save on our monthly expenses. Our out-of-pocket costs were actually $14,000 including some physical therapy and medications that weren't included.

10.3.3   Is a good hospital included in my plan?

The third issue in choosing a health plan is the hospital you might be using. This might be the most important decision of all. If you aren't tied at the hip to one doctor, you should choose your insurance plan that allows care at the best local hospital. Why? You might not even know the area of specialty and thus the doctor you might need (from arrhythmia care to a kidney transplant), so you want to make sure you choose a place known for great care.

How do you pick the best hospital? Of course, you look at TV ads or billboards. *No!* Do a little research.

Like many Top Doctor lists, most of the Best Hospital lists are not valuable because hospitals pay to get on them. In fact one local hospital administrator got caught receiving kickbacks (limo rides, nice hotel, and so on) from a hospital-rating program, which resulted in his termination. In my opinion, the only hospital rating agency with any credibility is *U.S. News & World Report.* Just like the college rankings, *U.S. News* has made a business of rating hospitals. Instead of high fees for consideration, *U.S. News* makes their money on ads they sell to those of us who go to their site to view the rankings.

To compare hospitals, they use a complex criteria that I think are categories of value to most of us:[6]

[6] Olmsted, Murrey G. et al. *Methodology: U.S. News & World Report Best Hospitals 2014-2015.* 2015.

- **Volume 30%** (remember how I said volume in physicians or hospitals matters a lot)

- **Outcomes 32.5%** (administrative speak for mortality rate)

- **Reputation 27.5%** (random survey of specialists in their area)

- **Patient safety 10%** (a valuable metric but the measurement is flawed)

After each category is the percentage weight of each category in the 2014-15 list. Other factors, such as other *key technologies,* are considered because the cardiac care is better if the hospital also has a well-rounded medical care service, just in case you need a lung or kidney specialist while there. The same goes for advanced technologies, which are required to make the list, such as advanced radiology and nuclear medicine services, transplant services, and the presence of a trauma center.

The reputation score is biased towards those with a medical school affiliation because we all vote for our alma mater and consider those teaching hospitals to be better. In my opinion, teaching does not always translate to better care because I would rather have an experienced doctor working on me instead of a trainee under supervision. However, the requirements to be a good teacher as well as the checks and balances necessary with a large institution do often translate into excellent care. Similarly, a reputation for basic science research does not always translate into great medical care. For research, you want an institution that does clinical research (on people, not rats) because they will provide access to the latest advances that might not be FDA-approved yet, such as the leadless pace-maker we will explain later.

In my opinion, one factor that is not weighted high enough by *U.S. News* is nursing care. There is now a separate national nursing survey, called Magnet Status, which is awarded only to those hospitals who truly value their nurses. The American Nurses Credentialing Center criteria measures outcomes, job satisfaction, low turnover, decision making, quality of care, and so on. Good nursing care translates into good overall medical care. Because only 6% of U.S. hospitals are awarded the Mag-net Status designation, keep this list in mind when picking a hospital.

Appropriately so, volume of patients cared for remains criti-cal in the *U.S. News* hospitals rankings because they won't even consider a cardiology program unless there are at least 1,335 cardiac patients and 500 surgeries a year. This alone narrows the more than 5,000 U.S. hospitals down to about 2,000.

For cardiac care, it is essential to align with a *local hospital* for emergent needs. Remember that an ambulance will gener-ally only take you to the nearest hospital, so it is often helpful to have a pre-existing relationship there. Of course, there is nothing wrong with shopping around the country for a com-plex procedure if your budget allows (and at least around your area finding one with volume and the other factors mentioned above). Just remember that aside from the procedure, follow-up care is challenging if your hospital is far from home. Just because the Cleveland Clinic is number one on the list, doesn't mean you need to get your treadmill in beautiful East Cleve-land.[7]

How do you use the *U.S. News* score? Go to the *U.S. News* hospital rankings website and choose: *Cardiology and Heart Surgery*. Enter your local hospitals and evaluate their relative rankings as a starting point in your search. Then, factor what is uniquely important to you and your family, whether that be other specialty care, the cost of the insurance at the number-one site, nursing care, free parking, and so on. You think I jest, but we have patients who transfer care when they learn they

[7] At age 22, I drove a U-Haul truck from California to New York headed to med school, the truck packed with everything in the world that I owned, pretty much a microscope and a lot of socks. In Cleveland, I stayed at a Howard Johnson's just off the freeway. When I got to my hotel room, I had a sickening feeling. Didn't I just park the truck there? Apparently, some bright crooks hung out in the hotel restaurant just waiting for a rental truck, because it would be pre-packed with belongings they could fence. They got mine. A couple of days later, my truck was found in a special part of Cleveland (use your imagination), but none of its contents were ever recovered. To this day, my family calls them the "blue sock gang" because we bet they still haven't run out of socks 40 years later.

have to pay $4 for parking. It's not necessary to choose a top-50 program out of the 5,000 hospital choices, but you should at least pick one that is well ranked.

10.4   Scripps

I must mention that Scripps Hospitals is ranked by *U.S. News* for cardiac care in the top 20 again this year, our third year in a row. I am proud of that accomplishment because we are not associated with a medical school, so our ranking should be lower on the reputation score. However, we are high volume and high quality. For example, we have five EP labs and are growing.

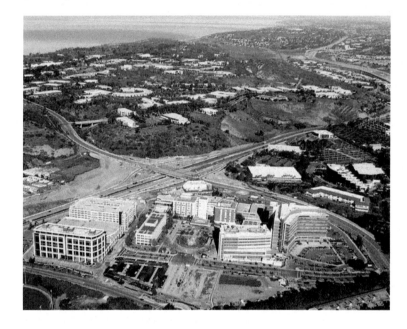

Figure 10.4: Aerial photo of Scripps La Jolla Campus (Photo by Fred Waller, Scripps Health).

In a program with 14 EP doctors and more than 100 cardiologists like ours, it is likely that there is a robust quality program to ensure proper care. We have also been designated a three-time Magnet Status nursing care award winner.

In terms of cardiology, Scripps has some of the finest doctors in the country, including:

- Eric Topol (from wireless health, genomics, and Cleveland Clinic fame)

- Paul Teirstein (interventional cardiology and transcatheter aortic valve replacement (TAVR) authority)

- Andrea Natale (part-time here but famous former Cleveland Clinic ablation doctor)

- Doug Gibson (the largest WATCHMAN™ implanter in the United States, just completing number 100)

- John Rogers (the first and one of the largest Medtronic Reveal LINQ™ implanters)

- Tom Heywood (international authority on heart failure)

- Brent Eastman (national founder of trauma surgery programs, former chief medical officer and former president of the American College of Surgeons)

- Chris Van Gorder (not a cardiologist but a famous hospital administrator, Scripps CEO, author, and past president of the American College of Healthcare Executives)

In 2015, we opened a new dedicated heart hospital, called the Scripps Prebys Cardiovascular Institute, attached to Scripps Memorial Hospital in La Jolla.

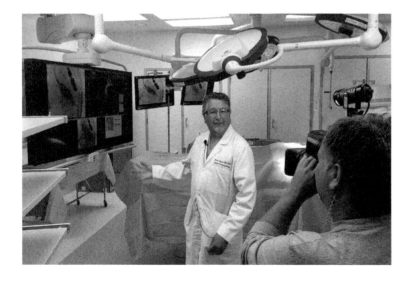

Figure 10.5: The author demonstrating one of the hybrid operating rooms for local TV in the new Scripps Prebys Cardiovascular Institute on opening day, March 8, 2015 (Photo by C. Van Gorder).

Combining two great programs, the cardiologists at Scripps Clinic have now joined us to add to our volume and expertise.

While a new hospital doesn't necessarily mean better care, it often does help.[8] The nurses, doctors, and all the staff are proud of our state-of-the-art facilities and that pride translates into a desire to provide the best care. In addition, patients love the beautiful private rooms with floor-to-ceiling windows that have views of La Jolla. It sure beats my medical school hospital, which had a lovely view of a cemetery from the ICU. At least the trip was short if they received what doctors call a "celestial discharge."

[8] You too can have your name on the next tower if you write a check for $100 million.

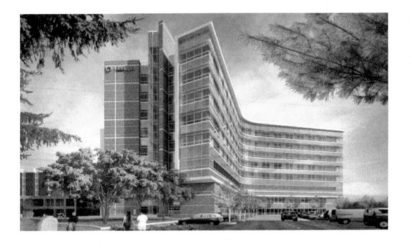

Figure 10.6: Scripps Prebys Cardiovascular Institute (With permission, Scripps Health).

10.5   Dealing with insurance companies

One of the true pioneers of cardiac EP, and an incredibly nice guy to boot, is Dr. David Cannom. David once had a simple slide in an arrhythmia lecture:

There are Only Three Treatments for Serious Arrhythmias

- Drugs

- Devices

- HMOs

He explained that when he prescribes a drug, an insurance company might counteract his choice. Similarly, when he recommends device surgery, this might be denied. So, "obviously,

HMOs have an alternative better treatment plan than I can recommend."

Let me digress and relate what happened recently in support of this often unnecessary roadblock to proper care. I saw a new patient in the office, a very nice but unfortunate man who had a massive heart attack at age 48. Four years later now, the scar from the heart attack has deteriorated his heart pumping function so that his ejection fraction (EF) has decreased from 55% (normal is 55% to 70%) to 37% to 33% to now 25% despite medication treatment. Based on the MADIT study previously mentioned, I recommended implantable cardioverter defibrillator (ICD) surgery. As you might recall, way back in 1996 this landmark study randomized high-risk patients between what then was conventional treatment vs. an implantable defibrillator (ICD). The ICD group had a 54% greater chance of living. All the major governing bodies in cardiology have since designated that this patient group is a *Class I, Level of Evidence A* indication, their highest level of recommendation, that defibrillator surgery is essential.

The new patient's HMO required a peer-to-peer consultation before approving admission for the procedure. Apparently, my dictated note and trained staff weren't adequate enough to get the authorization. They required that the implanting physician speak directly with the insurance company physician before authorizing payment (which won't come until at least a month after the surgery anyway). I called the HMO, got a recording, entered the patient's account number, and was transferred to an assistant who had several administrative questions for me.

After being placed on hold, I was eventually connected to the insurance company physician, who had no cardiology background. I explained the situation and fortunately, he promptly provided an authorization number, a lengthy 16-digit code to use for documentation purposes so we could get our patient scheduled. This went smoothly, but it still took about 20 minutes of my time.

In my opinion, this system is intentionally designed to delay approvals. These delays come at several steps in the process— before my staff learns of this insurance company's newest requirements, the possibility that I am too busy to call them promptly, the chance the phone gets disconnected (happens all too frequently), or an account number or authorization code gets transposed. Regardless, the surgery is then needlessly delayed. This delay has to translate into excessive preventable deaths but saves the insurance company money.

Don't get me wrong. There were many problems with the old type of unsupervised health care practice, not just from runaway costs. However, with current incentives, HMOs might be motivated to *delay* care. They do recognize that avoiding treatment for a slow lingering disease process like AIDS or breast cancer is bad for business. Those patient groups have clout with public forums and state insurance commissions. However, sudden death prevention that costs more than $50,000 per patient is a perfect target for what I call "malignant neglect." If the delay, or miscommunication, results in an avoidable sudden death, this is highly unlikely to translate into negative publicity or a lawsuit. From a cold-hearted bean counter's perspective, my patient's future lost insurance premiums will never compensate the insurance company for the cost of one $50,000 defibrillator admission. Thus, malignant neglect.

An appropriate new type of research now focuses on cost-effectiveness studies to compare one type of care with another.

For example, it has been shown that if you want the most bang for your buck, called cost per life-year saved, ICDs are cheaper than some treatments we take for granted (for example, kidney dialysis in the elderly). I certainly agree that scarce health care resources should be spent in a way that saves the most people for the longest time. This type of analysis has its benefits. We all agree that observation in the ICU is not necessary for a common cold, so we really do ration health care every day. With limited resources, it makes sense to use our health care dollars wisely. Unfortunately, if health care were actually a free market, too many would neglect traditional care and spend their dollars on supplements or a weekly massage. Thus, it isn't as simple as just letting the patient be in charge.[9]

Of course, I have no proof that insurance companies want customers to die but with quarterly profits and stock prices driving their rewards, their motivation might sometimes conflict with the patient's best interest. I have one powerful recommendation if you are ever in this situation, *be your own advocate.*

[9] The doctor gave me a bill and told me I had 6 weeks to live. I told him, "I can't pay this!" So he gave me 6 more.

10.6 Wrap

As we have discussed, it is important to find the doctor most suitable for you and your specific needs. That should include a PCP as well as a specialist. These days, patients with heart disease often have several specialists, such as cardiologists to treat coronary disease; electricians like me, cardiac EPs; heart failure specialists; and others. To determine the right team, it is usually best to start by finding the right hospital that fits with your insurance plan. Often, word-of-mouth recommendations are valuable. Still, do your homework and evaluate the doctor and hospital before committing to care.

These days navigating the health insurance system is critical to ensuring you can get to the people you need.

One of the most useful pieces of information for dealing with insurance companies in any capacity is, *be your own advocate*. The vocal patient, the "squeaky wheel," will often get an approval when the quiet nice guy will get denied. Insurance companies live in fear of complaints to the state insurance commission, so you can sometimes encourage them to do what is right by a gentle reminder of your power.

11

Blood thinners and prescription medications

In 1939, a pickup truck that a frustrated farmer named Ed Carlson was driving arrived unannounced at the Wisconsin Department of Agriculture. In it was a milk jug full of unclotted blood and in the back, another dead cow that he unceremoniously presented to Dr. Karl Paul Link and his colleagues. The jug of uncoagulated blood lying on the floor of Link's laboratory changed the course of history. Scientists recognized that these cows were bleeding to death from something they ingested in mold associated with damp sweet clover hay. It took until 1948 before warfarin could be isolated and synthesized and until 1954 for FDA approval.

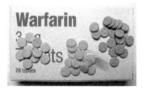

Figure 11.1: Multi-color warfarin tablets (Photo by GoneGone-Gone/Wikimedia).

Warfarin is named for the Wisconsin Alumni Research Fund, which funded the original veterinary research. For nearly 50 years, warfarin, brand name Coumadin®, has been the only blood thinner available by prescription and remains the most common to this day. To avoid turning out like that farmer's cows, the level of blood thinning needs to be frequently monitored with blood tests now called an International Normalized Ratio (INR); the previous warfarin test was called a ProTime.

Around the same time that warfarin was being promoted to the Food and Drug Administration (FDA) for human consumption, the same scientists sold warfarin as a rodenticide (that's scientist talk for "kills rats"). I don't understand why so many patients are concerned that their medicine is a rat poison; trust me, I'm a doctor. Here is some more information you will only get here: The reason warfarin works is that rats cannot vomit. Rats sample a new food and wait a short time to see if they become sick. Warfarin tricks them because its effects often

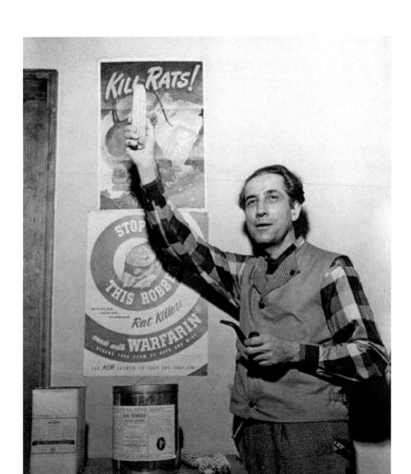

Figure 11.2: The co-developer of warfarin, Dr. Karl Link, demonstrating how it really is rat poison. I hope Karl remembered to put the pipe in his mouth and not the corn cob soaked in the poison (Photo courtesy Heart Rhythm Society Archives).

take days to occur and those little rat brains can't associate that tasteless pill they ate last week with the internal bleeding that happens. However, there is a reason rats will outlive humans after the apocalypse. The entire rat species has now developed immunity to warfarin. So exterminators have moved on to new rodenticides.

If you have an artificial valve or heart valve disease and atrial fibrillation (AF), warfarin remains the only drug approved for blood thinning. However, for most patients, such as those with AF, risk of leg clots and other needs, there now are many choices. Warfarin remains popular for several reasons:

- Cheapest by far (about $10 compared to up to $400 for the new drugs; that's a month)

- Blood can be monitored, even at home, for proper anticoagulation level

- Simple reversal agents abound, including vitamin K

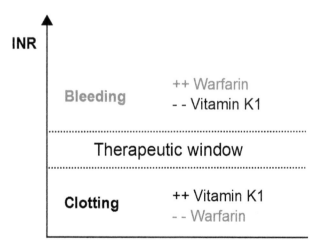

Figure 11.3: The therapeutic window of warfarin.

For many patients taking warfarin, it is literally a pain because they must get a needle stick every few weeks to monitor their blood thinning, the INR. These blood tests can be expensive too. For such a common drug, warfarin is quite dangerous with a narrow range of safety from your blood being too thin (ask Ed Carlson's cows about that) to too thick (so you remain unprotected from clotting or strokes).

The blood-thinning protection is especially dependent on intake of vitamin K foods, such as leafy vegetables.[1] Eat a salad with spinach, broccoli, or lettuce and your INR might drop because the vitamin K overwhelms your normal warfarin dose. On the opposite side, many medications, a gastrointestinal illness-producing diarrhea, or a diet low in vitamin K can all thin the blood to dangerous levels.

11.1 Novel Oral Anticoagulants (NOACs)

Anyone with a TV recognizes that there are some new blood thinners in town. After essentially providing no alternative since 1954, warfarin (Coumadin®) now has some competition. Called NOACs as a group, the "N" is for **N**ew or **N**ovel or maybe "**N**ot cheap" **O**ral **A**nti**C**oagulants, these drugs provide several advantages over that old-time rat poison. NOACs work differently than warfarin, which works on vitamin K necessary for certain clotting factors.

NOACs work on different parts of the coagulation cascade, such as inhibiting Factors Xa or IIa (no, there is not a quiz coming). Regardless of the factor, all these drugs work in similar ways inhibiting some of the clotting factors before harmful clots can form.

There are four NOACs on the market today, Eliquis®, Xarelto®, Pradaxa®, and Savaysa®.[2] These four NOAC drugs are pretty similar, though some are once a day, others twice a day, and some are safe if you have kidney disease, others are not, and so on. As a group, they have several advantages:

- No need to monitor blood for efficacy (more reliable thinning than warfarin, even with its blood INR monitoring)

- Fewer drug and food interactions (you can go back to eating spinach like Popeye)

- A more reliable metabolism with no blood tests needed

- Less brain bleeding complications, yet more stomach bleeding (which organ would you choose to preserve?)

- Faster acting. We used to keep people in the hospital for several days on intravenous heparin until oral warfarin provided protection.

[1] Popeye the Sailor Man was a popular cartoon from the 1950s where the hero would consume a can of spinach so that he would get strong enough to fend off his arch enemy, Bluto, and save his damsel in distress, Olive Oyl. With all that fighting, I guess it was good that Popeye's blood remained thick from all that spinach. The reason spinach was chosen for Popeye was its known high content of iron, a key ingredient for red blood cells.

[2] Did you know that companies routinely spend over $1 million for name consultants for new brands? They used to save money on names. In 1963, Southern Methodist University (SMU) was playing football against the University of Michigan. Ford VP Lee Iacocca visited the SMU locker room and told the team he was honoring their performance with his new car the Mustang. The two Mustang logos are identical except the horse runs to the right for SMU and to the left for the car.

- Faster clearing so reversing the blood thinner with another medicine might not be necessary when it's stopped

As the most interesting man in the world said, "I don't always take an anticoagulant, but when I do, it is a NOAC." However, there are also disadvantages to NOACs. Number one might be the cost, which is up to $400 if you don't have a prescription plan. In that case, warfarin would be best for you.[3] Also, there is not an easy antidote, comparable to vitamin K (or also fresh frozen plasma) for warfarin. One FDA antidote for Pradaxa®, Praxbind®, was just approved, but in the rare situation that you can't wait for the anticoagulant drug to clear, you can give prothrombin complex concentrate (PCC) to reverse the effects of any NOAC. Don't worry; remember that old medical adage, "All bleeding stops eventually."

[3] Remember Chevy Chase in *Caddyshack* talking to filthy Bill Murray? "We have a pond and a pool ... the pond would be best for you."

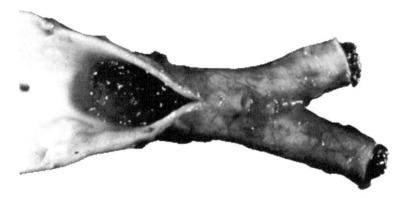

Figure 11.4: Obstruction of a blood vessel by a clot (Armed Forces Institute of Pathology).

Anticoagulants are most commonly prescribed for preventing stroke in AF but are also used in many other settings, such as clots in your legs, called deep venous thrombophlebitis or your lungs, called a pulmonary embolism. Strangely, the NOACs don't seem to work in preventing a stroke if your AF is due to a heart valve problem, such as those caused by rheumatic fever in childhood or in those who have already had heart surgery and have a mechanical valve. In the future, this might become less of a concern because rheumatic fever will vanish like smallpox has disappeared. Also, today heart surgeons are now using bioprosthetic valves, or tissue valves, instead of metal ones. Finally, with additional research, it is likely an instant NOAC reversal agent will be available soon.

In the meantime, stick with the rat poison if you have a valve problem and AF.

11.2   Aspirin

It is interesting to note the pendulum is swinging away from aspirin currently.

There seems to be no advantage of taking an antiplatelet agent, like aspirin, along with a NOAC; in fact, you just have more bleeding problems. For patients who do not take an oral anticoagulant, recent research suggests that taking nothing is just as good as taking a daily aspirin.

For garden-variety prevention of heart disease, the benefits of aspirin are quite small, such that the side effects (increased intestinal or brain bleeding) outweigh the benefits for those at low risk. Aspirin might cause even greater problems in those with diabetes.

Of course, if you are having a heart attack right now, chew (don't swallow) an aspirin, put this book down (pay for it first if you are at the bookstore), and call 911. If you have known heart disease, such as a prior heart attack, aspirin remains of benefit, probably. Ask your doctor.

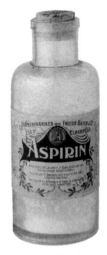

Figure 11.5: A bottle of Bayer Aspirin from 1899 (Photo by Bayer AG/Wikimedia).

11.3   Stopping your anticoagulant

One of my pet peeves is to get a message from a surgeon, "Please give clearance to stop our patient's blood thinner before surgery." Now, I am glad they ask, but surgeons love to overdo this request. You must understand where they are coming from. If you get a big bruise or blood loss from your surgery, the surgeon gets instantly blamed. If a blood transfusion is needed, the surgeon gets written up.

Unfortunately, if you have a stroke, they don't seem to associate that with having stopped your blood thinner.[4]

At the very least, NOACs should be stopped for no more than 24 to 48 hours in advance of surgery. However, it is becoming increasingly understood that stopping anticoagulation places patients at an even higher risk of stroke just from temporarily stopping the drug. Most EP doctors now do all their procedures (device surgery, ablations, and so on) without stop-

[4] A neighbor of mine had his NOAC stopped for a full week before a prostate operation (2 days is plenty, if at all). He had known AF with no prior strokes. The day after his surgery he had a big one. Two years later, he still requires around-the-clock care because he can't move his left side at all. His prostate isn't big anymore and he didn't bleed at surgery but his life is ruined. Make sure you have a very good reason to stop your blood thinner.

ping these anticoagulants at all. Even trying to "bridge" with an IV blood thinner like heparin or Lovenox® before surgery (in place of the oral drug) has been shown to be harmful due to excessive bleeding. Just take the darn anticoagulant and recognize that if you get a bruise, it will resolve and it certainly beats having a stroke. For many surgeries, there is now data that bleeding is no more likely to occur on the NOAC than off, so that bruise really was the surgeon's fault in the first place.

To be fair, some procedures are riskier than others, like open heart surgery and other major arterial procedures. I still recommend briefly stopping anticoagulants for these types of major surgeries. The rest of the time, I just tell the surgeon, "No."

11.4   Beta blockers

The most commonly prescribed heart medicine is a beta blocker. These drugs essentially block adrenaline (epinephrine), which can be very useful in slowing AF, preventing heart failure, lowering blood pressure, and many other scenarios—even stage fright or fear of flying! There are at least 20 beta blockers available by prescription, and that doesn't even count the anti-arrhythmics, some that also have beta-blocking properties, like sotalol and amiodarone. The most commonly prescribed beta blockers are Toprol-XL® or the generic metoprolol, Tenormin® or the generic atenolol and Coreg® or generic carvedilol. Although you will read about all sorts of side effects including fatigue and shortness of breath, give them a fair try when prescribed. They are the most commonly used heart drugs for a reason.

Although somewhat controversial, data suggests that you do better with any cardiac surgery if you take a beta blocker in advance, but probably not for noncardiac surgery (I told you it was controversial). Recently, a pacemaker patient decided to stop his atenolol for 3 days before a surgery without instruction. We had him take a pill with a sip of water before the surgery and he did great (what more proof do you need?). Open heart surgery patients are commonly pre-medicated with a beta blocker. Take your medicine before surgery (with a small sip of water) unless instructed to hold it.

I think it is reasonable to assume that the human animal was not designed for the daily stresses of life in the 21st century. Until we evolve in a way to better handle stress, beta blockers might have value for a host of problems from heart failure to hypertension to stage fright to migraines to angina to AF.[5]

[5] My doctor told me to avoid any unnecessary stress. So, I didn't open his bill.

11.5   Anti-arrhythmics

Numerous drug types are lumped into the term anti-arrhythmics. This actually does fit the rule that when you see a lot of drugs available for one problem, no one drug is really that exceptional.

Today, common drugs include flecainide, propafenone, sotalol, Multaq®, and amiodarone. Not uncommonly, patients with arrhythmias go from one to another in hopes of finding one that works. Often, none work. Now, I am a bit biased because if your arrhythmia is easily controlled on the first drug, you might never end up in my office. However, I often remind patients of the old commercial: "You can see me now, or you can see me later." Try an anti-arrhythmic, but you will likely be back later for an ablation.

Some older approved drugs are now being recycled as anti-arrhythmics. Ranexa®, an anti-anginal drug, might have anti-arrhythmic properties, commonly used in combination with Multaq®. Mexiletine, an old drug touted as oral lidocaine, has regained popularity. It might be a while before the FDA approves any new anti-arrhythmics.

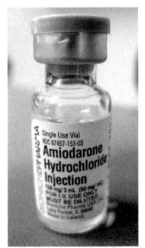

Figure 11.6: A single dose vial of Amiodarone HCL preparation for IV administration (Photo by Intropin/Wikimedia).

Between side effects and ineffectiveness, anti-arrhythmics are often *not* long-term solutions. Some have even been shown to make arrhythmias worse, called pro-arrhythmic (clever, eh?) and can lead to an *increased* risk of sudden death. The pharmaceutical manufacturers have recognized the risks of testing new anti-arrhythmic drugs; the FDA has approved only one in the last two decades.

11.5.1   Amiodarone

On a daily basis, I describe the anti-arrhythmic amiodarone (Cordarone®, Pacerone®) as the "best and the worst in one pill."

As we call it, "amio" has a strange history. In 1961, it was de-

veloped in Belgium to treat angina (chest pain). Fearful of the
FDA, the drug company never submitted for U.S. evaluation.
Serendipitously, heart doctors in South America and elsewhere
found that it appeared to control all types of arrhythmias. Word
of mouth and early publications suggested amio had no side
effects and almost always worked (both not true.) At the behest
of U.S. physicians, the FDA approved it here only for compas-
sionate use. Physicians in the arrhythmia world were placed
on special lists just to be able to prescribe it. It was almost like
ordering an illegal drug; it would come by mail from overseas
and could be provided free with certain limitations, essentially
unregulated by the FDA. Remember that at the time, we had no
ablation and few effective medications (still don't) for arrhythmia management.

By the early 1980s, some bizarre amiodarone side effects
emerged, so the FDA stalled approval. The drug company
threatened to stop providing it free to U.S. doctors until finally
in 1985 amio became FDA approved. However, its approval
came with one of the rare "black box" warnings about its risks.
It states that approval is only for "life-threatening arrhythmias
for which no other treatment is feasible."

Although commonly used for many arrhythmias, including AF, its use is actually off-label for that even today. Amazingly, many of the drugs we prescribe today for AF, including flecainide and sotalol are not FDA approved for that use
(even President Bush was on a drug not FDA approved for his
AF). Fortunately, U.S. physicians can prescribe an approved
medicine for other uses, though with increased medicolegal
liability. Today, amiodarone remains the most often prescribed
anti-arrhythmic agent accounting for about 25% of total pre-
scriptions.

The list of amiodarone side effects would take its own chapter. As it has a very slow onset, it is also slow to clear, lasting
a month or longer, so side effects might be difficult to treat.
The worst problem is pulmonary toxicity, a type of potentially
fatal lung scarring. It is estimated that 5 to 15% of patients
maintained on a dose of 400 mg or more daily develop this life-
threatening side effect. With the lower doses more commonly
used today, that number is less than 2%. Other common side effects include sunburn, corneal deposits, ataxia (incoordination),

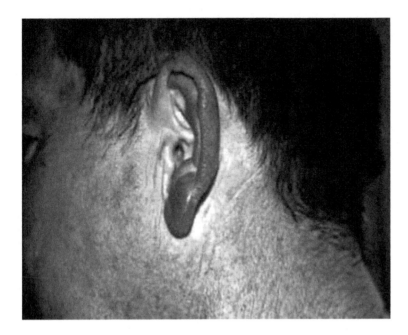

Figure 11.7: With long-term high doses, amiodarone deposits in the skin, especially on the face, causing a bluish-purple discoloration (Photo courtesy Heart Rhythm Society Archives).

liver damage, thyroid and skin toxicity, and so on.

If you aren't already frightened, take a look at the figure illustrating a patient with skin toxicity from amiodarone. I think the Blue Man Group must be on this drug. Amiodarone is the best and worst wrapped up in one.

11.5.2 Digoxin

Digoxin (Lanoxin®) is on its last legs. Extracted from the foxglove plant in the late 1700s, digoxin was touted as treatment for dropsy. When was the last time you saw a good case of dropsy? Actually, dropsy—today called heart failure—is still the number-one condition requiring hospitalization in the new millennium.

If digoxin was so effective for dropsy, how come it is still a problem? Brilliant, Sherlock. Recent research shows that digoxin provides no benefit at all and potential harm for heart failure (or dropsy).

Every research study now seems to show a new problem for digoxin. It appears to rarely be of any benefit in treating AF either. One study reviewing data from the huge AFFIRM trial on more than 4,000 patients found a 41% greater chance of dying, even when adjusted for other factors. After its benefit for heart failure was debunked, digoxin was touted to help control rapid AF heartbeat rates. However, it only works at rest, not with exercise, when rapid rates are more likely to occur. With digoxin, the safety window is very small; it doesn't take much of an overdose to knock people off.[6] Unlike amio, perhaps we should just call digoxin "the worst and worst in one pill." Perhaps it's time to put digoxin and the foxglove plant back in the hen house. Of course, check with your doctor before stopping any medication.

[6] Remember that male nurse in 2013 who killed 40 hospital patients in New Jersey? This so-called "angel of mercy" used intravenous digoxin as his poison.

11.6   Pain medications

As you know, we have a national problem with narcotic addiction. A decade ago, we were told that physicians were cruel, inadequately treating pain due to insufficient doses and frequency of prescription narcotics. As a result, usage of narcotics like OxyContin or Vicodin increased for legitimate pain, but they are incredibly addictive. Eventually, the doctor won't renew a prescription and the addicted patient turns to illegal drugs like heroin. Heroin use has jumped 60% in the past decade. Today, the new heroin addict is far more commonly a non-Hispanic Caucasian in their 20s to 40s living in the suburbs. Heroin use is decreasing for non-whites.

Addicted patients' friends or family even smuggle narcotics into hospitals. I recall one patient whose girlfriend would use his IV to inject him with heroin. A clever doctor added an ampule of the narcotic reversal agent, Narcan, to each IV bag so that the heroin did not have the desired effect.

Nurses and physicians using illegal prescription narcotics is a problem too. One local San Diego company, Pyxis, has come up with a medication-locking system, now in use in many hospitals, to document who administers which drug.

Narcotics are obviously valuable for treating severe pain. However, I rarely ever prescribe them for outpatient use. Although expensive, intravenous acetaminophen is growing in popularity in the hospital because it is far more potent than the oral version and much safer than narcotics. Over-the-counter drugs like acetaminophen, aspirin, and the non-steroidal

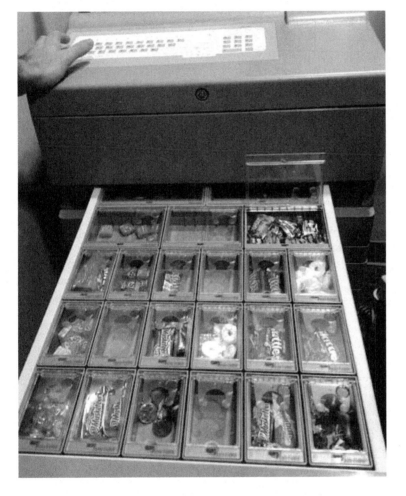

Figure 11.8: Pyxis medication locking system used in a hospital where Skittles addiction is apparently a big problem. I'm not sure they are delivering the right message about drug addiction (With permission, Thomas Stritter, RN).

anti-inflammatories (NSAIDs), such as Advil or Aleve, are often great pain relievers. Even ice on a wound will help with pain. No one ever got addicted to ice (unless it was with their Scotch). Which reminds me, don't mix alcohol and calculus, it's bad to drink and derive.

11.7   Wrap: Always take your medicine

Here's another lesson from mom. One of the most dramatic examples of not taking your medicine involved NCAA superstar Hank Gathers, the number-one NBA draft prospect in 1990 who led the nation in scoring and rebounding.

While still in college at Loyola Marymount, Gathers collapsed at the free-throw line, awakened, and was subsequently diagnosed with a rare arrhythmia, exercise induced polymorphic ventricular tachycardia (PVT). In 1990, implantable cardioverter defibrillators (ICDs) were still new, so Gathers was first put on medications. He was prescribed the first beta blocker, Inderal. On game days, Hank felt fatigued from the drug, a common side effect especially with the first generation beta blockers. Much like any young kid, he felt invincible and just stopped taking his medicine on game days.

A couple of months later, during a televised game with Portland University, Gathers scored 8 points in the first few minutes, getting a high-five at half court. Suddenly, he collapsed, rising up only to slump back to the floor never to recover.

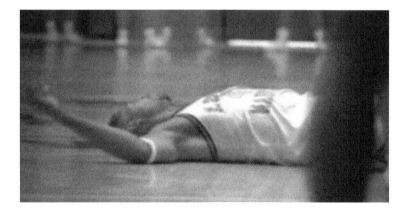

Figure 11.9: Hank Gathers of Loyola Marymount collapses after a dunk on March 4, 1990 (Screenshot).

At half court and live on national TV, Gathers died, without an attempt at defibrillation or even bystander CPR (this is why CPR is so important). Viewed in today's world, this delay is inconceivable. Paramedics arrived about 10 minutes too late. No one knows if Gather's PVT would have been prevented if he had taken his medication. He most certainly would have lived with prompt defibrillation, either from an ICD or an automatic external defibrillator (AED) at courtside. What a shame and a sad loss.[7]

Out of the subsequent publicity, substantial awareness has been raised about heart conditions. Many other athletes and non-athletes now recognize the need to take their prescription medicines. Today, some players in both college and professional sports play with implanted defibrillators. Recent research suggests that sudden death is no more likely to occur at athletic events than in other scenarios. However, anywhere a large group of people congregate, it is nice to have an AED available (I carry one in the trunk of my car).

We all like to think that it won't happen to us, especially when we're young. If you have a known condition, follow mom's advice and always take your medicine.

[7] Couturie, Bill. *ESPN 30 for 30: Guru of Go*, 2010. http://espn.go.com /30for30/film?page= guru-of-go.

12

Devices 1: So you need a pacemaker

First of all, do you really need a pacemaker? If a doctor has recommended a pacemaker, the answer is yes, you probably need a pacemaker.

When patients come for a second opinion about whether they need a device, unlike most second opinions, they usually leave with the same advice—get it done.[1]

Let's review the indications for a pacemaker; *indications* is the term physicians use for reasons a treatment is necessary. Most all are based on documented heart rhythm abnormalities like those we've discussed.

The most basic concept: *pacemakers* fix slow heart rhythms whereas *defibrillators* treat both slow and fast.

[1] Sometimes I tell the patient, "I think it's your heart but if you want a second opinion, I will say it's your lungs."

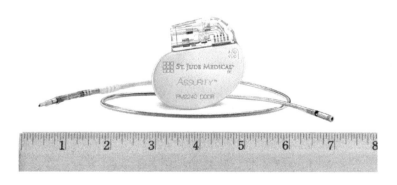

Figure 12.1: A typical permanent pacemaker and lead (With permission, St. Jude Medical).

The gold standard for knowing you need a pacemaker is to have an abnormally slow rhythm recording at the same time you have your intermittent symptoms, whether those are fainting, almost fainting, dizziness, chest pain, and others. Typically, a heart rate below 30 or a pause more than 3 seconds along with symptoms is considered an indisputable reason for a pacemaker.

Of course, we are not always able to document this safely. I recently heard about a patient who had three severe fainting episodes in 3 days. After the third time, he hit his head so hard, he needed to come to the ER for stitches and a CT scan. While there and fortunately lying on a gurney, he suddenly developed another episode of near-fainting at the same time a doctor observed his heart rhythm to be in the 30s. He received a permanent pacemaker without any problems and has never fainted since.

This story would have a happy ending except that the pacemaker patient sued his implanting doctor saying he never needed the pacemaker. Some stupid lawyer encouraged the whole thing. This attorney paid for the whole lawsuit himself hoping to get a large percentage of the settlement, called contingency. Of course, after more than a week in trial, the jury decided the patient really did need a pacemaker. The poor doctor went through hell just to spare his name in court. In California, a doctor's malpractice carrier still has to pay for all the doctor's legal expenses, even when the doctor wins.

In 2008 and 2012, copious guidelines sanctioned by all the major governing bodies in cardiology were published listing appropriate reasons to get a pacemaker. Although the documents are more than 75 pages each, and really boring, they can be distilled into these points:

- **Gold standard reasons you need a pacemaker**

  - Heart rate below 30 documented at the same time you have symptoms

  - Heart pauses more than 3 seconds or more while you have symptoms

- **Silver standard reasons you need a pacemaker (you still likely need one)**

  - Heart rate above 30 but below 45 at the same time you have symptoms

- Heart rate below 30 or pauses more than 3 seconds with symptoms but no EKG proof

- Repeated fainting spells presumed to be due to slow heart rates but not proven

- Third (complete) atrial valve block with heart rates 40 or below (even if no symptoms)

- **Bronze standard reasons you need a pacemaker (you might still need one)**

  - First- or second-degree AV block with symptoms

  - Bifascicular block (a type of bundle branch block) with symptoms

All of the above reasons for pacemakers should have the caveat "unless a reversible cause is present." If you have taken a medication that could have slowed your heart excessively, or even worse, overdosed on a medication, it makes sense to evaluate after the medicine has cleared, if safe. In this situation, sometimes a temporary pacemaker is needed.

Sometimes, other problems like an abnormal thyroid, heart attack, temporary catheter, or surgical injury to the conduction system can be a reason to wait to make sure the problem does not resolve on its own.

Unfortunately, many dangerously slow heart rhythms occur infrequently, so just because you stopped your eye drops and your heart is no longer slow, it is likely the problem will recur, and potentially at a bad time. Fainting is bad anytime but especially if you are driving a car, swimming, or in a situation where a fall could cause severe injury, such as head trauma. Clinical judgment needs to apply in such situations; normal people call this common sense. If you're fainting and it's putting you in danger, see a doctor.

12.1   *Causes of slow heart rates warranting a pacemaker*

There are innumerable causes for slow heart rates bad enough to warrant the need for a pacemaker. However, the number-one cause is simply growing old. Unfortunately, our electrical conduction system to the heart is similar to our hearing; it often wears out before we do. This has fancy names like Lev's disease, Lenegre's syndrome, idiopathic (a medical term for "cause unknown") fibrosis, or calcification of the heart's conduction system. Regardless, your heart's watch needs a new battery.

Sinus node disease and conduction problems are more common as we age. In fact, the average age for patients getting a pacemaker is older than 77. The oldest patient I have ever implanted a pacemaker in was 101. She (only women live past 100 for good reason) was still living independently and otherwise healthy and continues to do well at 103. A pacemaker, like a hearing aid, can make you functional again, ready to get back into the dating pool, or at least the shallow end.

Other common causes for needing a pacemaker besides age-related deterioration include:

- Born with third-degree heart block (congenital complete heart block)

- Heart also beats too fast and it can't be controlled without excessive slowing

- Developed heart block (not just artery blockage) at time of a heart attack

- Heart failure and evidence for abnormal pumping (called dyssynchrony)

- Recurrent fainting from low blood pressure that can't be controlled with medication

- Conduction system damaged during an auto accident, open heart surgery, or ablation procedure

- Getting an implantable cardioverter defibrillator (ICD) that comes with pacing (for free!)

- Certain viruses or parasites infecting the conduction system

- Other bad bugs (Lyme disease, spider bites, not just black widows)

- Drugs that permanently damage the heart (such as cocaine, ecstasy, or methamphetamines)

12.2   Types of pacemakers

Let's assume that you are convinced that you need a pacemaker. What kind should you get? Of course, your doctor will guide you with this, but I'll explain the basic types.

All pacemakers work about the same. A tiny electrical current is delivered to remind the heart cells to beat. The pacemaker does not make muscles beat, it just reminds them that it is past time for them to beat on their own. Imagine that they have a little alarm clock going off every second because once a second is a common pacemaker's set rate of 60 bpm. If the pacer does not sense the beating during that second, it delivers a small electrical pulse, typically 1 to 2 volts for just 1/2 of a millisecond. If you touch the pacemaker wire as it paces, you can't even feel it.

Fortunately, most heart cells, no matter how sick, can still respond to this alarm clock. Only when the heart has entirely given up, such that you need a heart transplant, is it necessary to provide more than this little electrical pulse to make it work again at the correct rate.

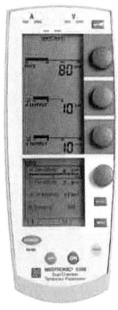

12.2.1   Temporary pacemaker

As noted, sometimes there is reason to believe that heart slowing will go away, so a temporary pacemaker is inserted. This is essentially a stiff wire inserted in a large vein in the neck attached to an external pacemaker box.

In recent years, temporary pacemakers have fallen into disfavor due to the risk of damage from the stiff wire and/or dislodgement.

Today, if it is likely that a permanent pacemaker will be needed, it is often done urgently so that you don't even require a risky temporary pacemaker. Or, if it is really unclear if a permanent device will be needed, a safer, soft permanent lead is inserted, externalized, and attached to a generator, though this can get expensive.

Figure 12.2: A typical temporary pacemaker box that attaches to the lead (With permission, Medtronic).

12.2.2   One-lead pacemakers

The very first pacemakers just paced in one location, typically the right ventricle to make the heart's pumping chambers pump faster. Not only did these giant pacemakers keep you alive, but each one came with a 24/7 nurse.

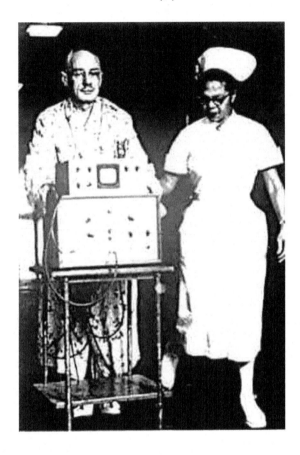

Figure 12.3: One of the first permanent pacemaker systems, allowing for the patient to ambulate (Photo courtesy Heart Rhythm Society Archives from work of Dr. Paul Zoll, circa 1955).

Since that photo taken in 1955 or so, pacemakers have gotten a lot smaller and no longer come with individual nurses. Nursing hats have also come a long way.

A one lead pacemaker is called a single-chamber device, which today is implanted in the lower chambers about 98% of the time. Most commonly, these are for people who have permanent AF, so a lead in the upper chambers wouldn't help anyway. Another reason for just implanting a single-chamber pacemaker is in patients who need pacing so rarely that one lead alone is adequate.

Today, with improved understanding, single-chamber pacemakers comprise a relatively small portion of pacemaker implants, about 10%, particularly in countries like the United

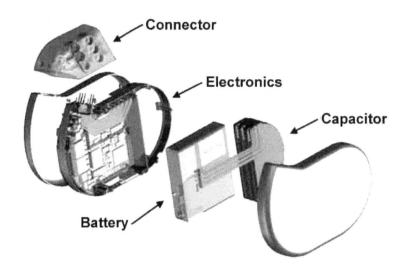

Figure 12.4: Components of a typical permanent pacemaker or defibrillator (With permission, Sanjeev Saksena, MD).

States where rationing of care has yet to become commonplace.

In France, for example, each hospital gets an annual budget to cover both pacemakers and defibrillators, usually less than the previous year's budget. The hospital might run out of funds earmarked for implanted devices by September. So, all year long, doctors will prescribe the cheaper single-chamber devices to save money for those cases later in the year.

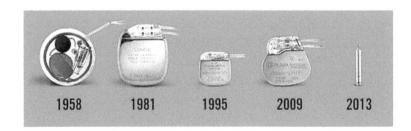

Figure 12.5: Evolution of pacemaker technology (With permission, St. Jude Medical).

12.2.3 Two-lead pacemakers

By far and away the most common pacemaker today is the dual-chamber pacemaker, comprising more than 50% of all implants today. Dual pacemakers have two separate leads, one that goes to the right atrium and one to the right ventricle.

Dual pacemakers more closely simulate the normal heartbeat that starts in the high-right atrium and courses down to the

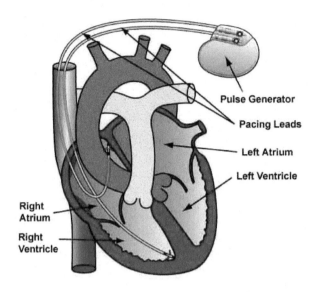

Figure 12.6: A drawing of the heart chambers showing typical locations for dual pacemaker leads in the right atrium and ventricle (Modified with permission af-ablation.org).

ventricles. These are amazingly smart machines that use two alarm clocks to figure out which chamber, or both, needs to be reminded to beat.

In addition, they restore the normal atrial beats first followed by the ventricles, A then V. This is called AV synchrony and can be associated with a 25% or greater improvement in heart pumping efficiency when pacing. Many people who get just a single-chamber pacer can get pacemaker syndrome where the loss of A then V timing makes them fatigued. The resumption of the more normal AV synchrony with a second pacing lead in the atrium is usually needed to resolve this issue. Despite using two leads, the dual-chamber pacemaker uses hardly more battery life than a single; the typical pacemaker today lasts 8 to 12 years.

12.2.4   Three-lead pacemakers

I'll bet you realized the next type is a triple-chamber pace-maker. The co-inventor of the ICD, Morty Mower, also invented the triple-chamber pacemaker.

I attended a medical meeting in Nice, France, (which indeed is very nice) in 1996. I bumped into Morty and he was all excited about this new concept of pacing both the right and left ventricles simultaneously to help the heart beat more synchronously. Knowing Morty, I figured this was another of his hair-brained ideas and that you can only win the lottery once and he'd already saved a gazillion lives by inventing the ICD. Flash forward a few years and the company Morty worked with invited me to participate in a trial where we would put wires on both the left and right ventricles. I agreed though I remained skeptical.

My very first *biventricular* pacemaker/defibrillator patient was a fascinating guy. "Lou" flew out from Louisiana just to be a trial subject for this new research opportunity. He was already on a heart transplant waiting list and was looking for other options. After discussing his options he agreed to pacemaker surgery on his open heart rather than replacing the one he had. A heart surgeon and I sewed a permanent pacing lead to the outside of his left ventricle, adapted it to a traditional dual-chamber pacemaker/defibrillator system with a simple Y connector for the two ventricular leads to work simultaneously as one.

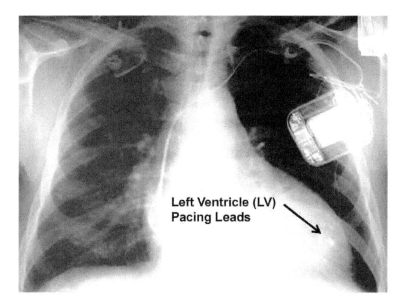

Figure 12.7: Actual chest x-ray of Lou, the first patient to get left ventricular epicardial pacing leads for cardiac resynchronization therapy (With patient permission).

Any electrician would appreciate the simplicity. Almost immediately, Lou felt dramatically better, even removing his name from the heart transplant waiting list. I was skeptical, but many of the subsequent research patients had similar amazing benefits.

About 6 months later, Lou flew back from Louisiana for a research follow-up visit and in his charming Southern accent said, "I feel like crap." He even nearly fainted in a San Diego restaurant the night before his office visit. I thought that the benefits from Morty's invention might be short-lived. Fortunately, I was wrong. When Lou came to the office, I found that one of his leads sewn on the outside of the left ventricle had broken. His heart rate was fine because he still had a dual system but he had lost the pacing synchrony of the right and left ventricles working together.

In those early days, we sewed a spare lead on the heart, just in case this happened, so re-attaching another left ventricular lead was simple. After resynchronizing his heart by reattaching the functioning left ventricular lead, Lou almost immediately felt great again. To me, this was better than any double-blind study to prove that this new biventricular pacing really worked. Of course, since then there have been numerous scientific studies espousing the advantages of biventricular pacing with fun names like PATH-CHF, MUSTIC, MIRACLE, CONTAK-CD (I was the lead author of this one), COMPANION, and CARE-HF.

A final note about Lou. As mentioned, he got off the transplant list and felt so good he went back to Louisiana, regularly playing golf with his 14-year-old son. One day, Lou got the first hole-in-one of his life and was so appreciative that he sent me the hole-in-one trophy.

Like many physicians, I have a bookshelf of mementos I've gathered over the years with awards and thank yous from grateful patients. Mine includes a few Best Doctor plaques, a Pioneer in the Field of Implantable Defibrillators award, and other artwork, but the hole-in-one trophy is by far my most prized keepsake.

12.2.5   *Cardiac resynchronization therapy (CRT)*

Triple-chamber pacing is now called cardiac resynchronization therapy (CRT) and also more commonly, biventricular pacing.[2] Even though the ventricles might be scarred or damaged differently in different patients, it is amazing to see that many

[2] Medical school rule number one appears again to keep you confused.

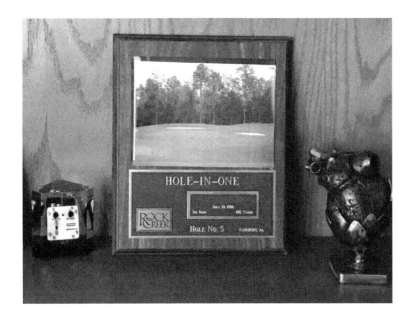

Figure 12.8: My prized hole-in-one trophy a patient sent me after he improved following biventricular pacing for heart failure (With patient permission).

patients benefit substantially from the relatively simple concept of adding another pacing lead to the left ventricle, pioneered by Dr. Mower.

Triple-chamber pacing really does resynchronize the heart in many patients, even reversing prior damage.

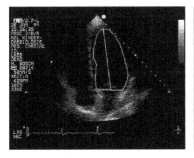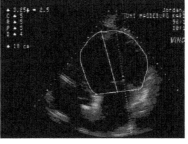

Figure 12.9: Still images from cardiac echos (ultrasound). The diseased heart (right) is markedly enlarged and ejects only 15% of its volume with each heartbeat.

The images shown are still frames from a movie of a standard echocardiogram (cardiac ultrasound) of two different patient's hearts. The one on the left has its left ventricle outlined in yellow. Imagine the movie that shows the heart squeezes with each beat, shortening in length and width with each heart-beat. The echo of the heart on the right shows that this patient's left ventrical is much larger, dilated from weakness, called a dilated cardiomyopathy. To make matters worse, if you saw the echo movie, you would realize this has a "beach ball effect" where it beats so poorly that one wall moves in while another moves out. This doesn't help blood pump out to where it is needed. As you can see, the ejection fraction (EF) is normal at 65% on the left but just one-fourth of that with the cardiomy-opathy on the right, down to 15%.[3] It isn't hard to figure out why this patient is always tired.

[3] Remember that ejection fraction (EF) equals the amount of blood pumped out with one heartbeart.

This could have been Lou. After his surgery, Lou's EF im-proved to about 30% just with CRT. That amount of improve-ment was enough to let him lead a normal life and get back to golfing with his teenage son.

Numerous research studies have shown that CRT can im-prove the EF an average of more than five points from 15% to 20%, though sometimes 30% or more as happened with Lou. Now, that might not sound like much, but the average CRT re-sponder improves more than one New York Heart Association (NYHA) class in functional capacity. In English, this improve-ment changes the patient's life. Instead of being homebound from fatigue and heart failure, the patient can now go shopping or play with the grandkids. Echo studies have found *reverse remodeling*, a fancy term to explain that these enlarged hearts shrink back closer to normal size. All just by adding a third pacing lead. Thanks, Morty (Dr. Mower).

You might be saying, if it gives people more energy, I want one of these! Unfortunately, it only works in selected patients. Here are the accepted criteria for CRT today (you need all three):

- Symptoms from heart failure (measured by NYHA func-tional class II or higher)

- Symptoms persist despite proper heart failure medication therapy

- Wide QRS on EKG, most commonly associated with a left bundle branch block

Another recent trial, called BLOCK-HF (doctors love these

cute acronyms) used triple-chamber pacemakers in everyone who needed pacing for every beat, such as those with complete heart block and found a benefit even if the baseline EF was almost normal (EF of 50% or less; normal is 55% or higher). CRT might help some with only mild heart failure too, so-called NYHA functional class I. We proved this in MADIT-CRT as well—that biventricular pacing can prevent weakened hearts from getting weaker and ever developing more severe heart failure.

The current teaching is to receive a triple-chamber CRT device if you will need pacing most of the time regardless of your EF or you have a pre-existing bundle branch block and a low EF, regardless of symptoms. If you pace rarely or you don't meet these criteria, a single- or dual-lead system is sufficient.

A quick commercial timeout. At Scripps, we were fortunate to implant the second transvenous CRT system in the world (conveniently, I don't remember who did the first).

The figure shows me and my team performing the operation. Today, this procedure is done more than 10,000 times a year around the world.

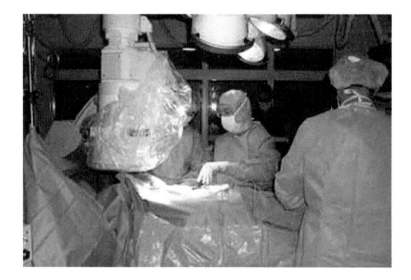

Figure 12.10: The second CRT in the world performed at Scripps (With patient permission).

12.2.6   Four-lead pacemakers

Kidding. There's no such thing. Yet. We stop at three today because both atria work fine together with just one lead.

12.3   Leadless pacemakers

In more than 50 years of development, the permanent pacemaker shrunk in weight from 300 grams to 30 grams. Nevertheless, the standard pacemaker today has many limitations, as I highlighted in a medical article in 2014:[4]

- Generator is remote from the heart

- Requires intravascular leads

- Frequent pocket-related concerns: discomfort, infection, hematoma

- Frequent lead-related concerns: Mechanical failures from movement, subclavian crush, lead-on-lead injury, challenges with removal

- Patient-perceived limitations: cosmetic concerns, disfigurement, mobility restrictions, MRI compatibility, travel restrictions, postoperative wound care, self-perception concerns, size, product recalls

- Physician concerns: radiation exposure, follow-up demands, technical challenges, reimbursement challenges, MRI compatibility

> [4] Higgins, Steven L. and Rogers, J.D. "Advances in pacing therapy. Examining the potential impact of leadless pacing therapy." *Innovations in Cardiac Rhythm Management,* 5:1825-1833, 2014.

As mentioned, the Achilles' heel of pacemakers are the leads; they move with every heartbeat and wear out. They can fracture under the collarbone when stretching your arm. The leads use electricity and they can be difficult to remove, sometimes requiring a complex laser-lead approach.

Wouldn't it be great if we didn't need them? Both St. Jude Medical and Medtronic have developed a revolutionary alternative, the leadless pacemaker, already the recipient of numerous innovation awards. These miniaturized devices have been technologically possible only recently because circuits and batteries have never been small enough for this approach. Until recently, the smallest pacemaker was still the size of a silver dollar, mostly battery because the electricity needed to travel down the lead required a certain size to last a reasonable time (10 years or so).

Just in the last few years pacemakers have shrunk another order of magnitude, down to 2 grams and less than 1 cc in size due to advances in technology.

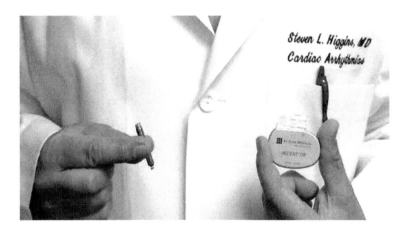

Figure 12.11: The leadless Nanostim™ pacemaker compared to a standard pacemaker generator.

These advances are a result of recent battery advances, low current communications, integrated circuits that no longer need to be flat (rolled in this device), and smaller batteries (less current) required by pacemakers closer to the heart. Amazingly, estimates are for these batteries to last about 15 years, 50% longer than the typical 10-year traditional pacemaker battery life.

Leadless, about the size of a cigarette butt (not that you would know what that is) are installed inside the heart, with a large screw that adheres to the wall of the right ventricle. Along with the technology, the delivery process took some cues from the space program.

As shown, after securing the tip in the heart muscle, the delivery system is undocked but attached with tethers for testing. Next, the tethers are carefully removed to leave the device in the heart, reminding it to beat at the programmed rate just like traditional pacemakers.

At their current stage, these leadless pacemakers have some disadvantages, most importantly the fact that they can only

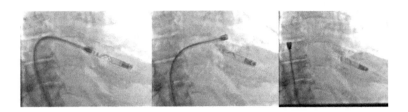

Figure 12.12: The delivery sheath first attached to the leadless pacemaker. Then, the sheath is untethered leaving the pacemaker in the right ventricle.

function as a single-chamber device and thus are helpful in only a small subset of those needing pacemakers today. Implants are limited to patients who have symptomatic bradycardia and:

- Have permanent atrial fibrillation (AF) and thus don't need atrial pacing

- Have sinus rhythm but a low level of activity or a short expected lifespan (but at least 1 year)

- Have sinus rhythm but only infrequent prolonged pauses

However, never fear, future advances are not far away with prototypes already available that can pace in two, and perhaps, three chambers just like pacemakers with leads. While still experimental in the United States, leadless pacemakers are available now in Europe and hopefully will be FDA approved by late 2016. In 10 years, it's likely most devices will be leadless, similar to these early ones.

12.4   Pacemaker brands

The investment to develop and gain regulatory approval is a huge hurdle. Thus, there are only a small number of companies that sell pacemakers and defibrillators to physicians and hospitals. I did hear of one stolen ICD listing on eBay, but normally, you need a doctor to prescribe it and a hospital to procure a device.

In approximate order of sales, the U.S. companies are Medtronic, St. Jude Medical, Boston Scientific, Biotronik, and Sorin-ELA.

That's it. Some physicians rotate their product selection in random order to be fair. The majority of us have a favorite company based on sales and service support, unique product features, ease of use, or whether the representative will bring lunch. Because there are differences in the tools necessary to implant different brands, it is generally not wise to request that your doctor implant a brand not used regularly. In addition, evaluation in the office requires programming a complex computer, which is unfortunately entirely different with each brand. It is difficult to have equal expertise with all five companies. In short, leave the brand selection to the expert; a full stomach leads to successful surgery.[5]

Complex medical devices go through a predictable product lifespan. When first developed, there are huge differences as some companies lead the process, others follow or wait to acquire the winners. New valuable features are added, leapfrogging the prior products on the market to make each company competitive. Then, as the product matures, advances become trivial. This stage of relative product equivalence results in a price war. If everything is essentially the same, called product parity, the basic discriminator is price. That is where we are today in the markets for pacemakers, defibrillators, and CRT devices. The products are very similar, though of course you would never get a manufacturer to agree with that statement.

If you step back and look at the device market, huge advances come once every 20 years—the pacemaker in 1960, the first defibrillator in 1980, the first CRT in 2000. We are getting dangerously close to 2020 with no huge advance on the horizon. I have enough experience to recognize that just before these other advances, no one predicted them either. I sure hope some genius is working on a great device-based health advance for 2020.

[5] True story: A sales rep for one of the device companies living in Naples, Italy, had his car stolen. In the trunk were five pacemakers and defibrillators for a local hospital. The rep knew that his company would fire him for losing the devices. He approached someone he was told was a local Mafia Don and cautiously explained that the medical devices had no market for resale. He added that if he didn't get them back, he would lose his job and his family would go hungry. The Mafia Don said he'd see what he could do. When the dejected salesman returned home, he found the five boxes sitting on his front doorstep undamaged. Who says the Mafia doesn't have a conscience?

12.5   Pacemaker replacements and upgrades

One of the gruesome facts of my specialty is the knowledge that many pacemaker or defibrillator patients won't outlive their device. Pacemakers typically last 8 to 12 years and ICDs 5 to 7 years.

Of course many patients do live long enough to need a new generator. We call it a battery change, but unlike your flashlight, replacing the battery doesn't work. We replace the entire unit, called a generator, usually without the need to change the leads. Often, generator changes are routine procedures and patients go home from the hospital the same day.

The only moving part of a device is the leads, moving up to 100,000 times a day with each heartbeat. So, leads do fail in a less predictable fashion than generators or batteries and sometimes need to be removed or replaced. If you ever need to have a lead removed, make extra sure your doctor has a lot of experience, because just like spouses, removing one is far more difficult the older they get. In the first few months after insertion, leads can be easily removed. After that, the body scars them down and removal might require a complex laser lead procedure to free them. Laser lead extraction is an expensive procedure, usually done by EP doctors in a cardiac surgery operating room because when things go wrong, they happen quickly. Fortunately, most leads can be safely extracted, or if not infected, abandoned without significant risk.

When you need a battery or generator change, it is useful to ask your physician if there is anything new to consider. More than 50% of my current generator changes actually get leads upgraded at that time, most commonly with the addition of a left ventricle lead to improve cardiac function with CRT. Just like with your car, as long as you have the engine open, you might as well change the gaskets too.

With reoperation, the biggest risk is infection. Inserting a foreign body like a pacemaker does not often result in infection the first time, less than 1% at most centers. However, at generator change time, that risk increases to more than 5%, more than 1 in 20. A pacemaker pocket is mostly scar tissue; one tiny bacterium might safely multiply there free from removal from the body unlike healthy tissue, where white blood cells mobilize to clean up our messes.

Device infections can be a huge problem, particularly in the patient who is dependent on the device to remain alive. In that situation, we commonly insert a clean new device on the other side (usually the right if the original was on the left) and then, only after it is done, sealed and protected, open the infected one and remove it. After you rid the body of the infected hardware, it commonly heals quickly.

By the way, although this work can be life-saving, most patients just care about the scar because that is all they can see. At reoperation, patients often joke about, "Why didn't you put in a zipper the first time?" I actually had one patient who tattooed a zipper around his scar. This wasn't so hilarious for me because when I did his generator change it took a lot of extra time to make sure the zipper lined up straight.

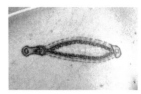

Figure 12.13: Everyone's a comedian: A zipper tattoo placed around a pacemaker scar making reoperation more challenging (With patient permission).

Another woman with a large device scar, posted her own tattoo on the Internet, apparently commissioned to distract you from the scar. As a device surgeon, my first thought on seeing her photo was who left that ugly scar (the mouth) on this pretty young woman? I would be run out of southern California if my work looked like that. Perhaps she could have used the money she spent on the tattoo and spent it on a better surgeon. At least she has a good sense of humor.

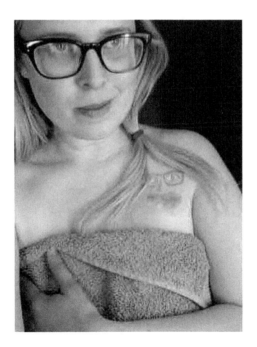

Figure 12.14: Don't be afraid to ask your doctor to "make it pretty" (With permission, B. Spinner).

Although the risks of lead movement are higher, in those who are self-conscious about appearance, I often put the pacemaker scar and device in the left armpit or along the breast and hide the device under it. I have even had some women ask if I can put a second device on the other side to balance the breasts (no). Fortunately, in La Jolla, we have talented plastic surgeons on every street corner who can help with that. No one wants to wear turtlenecks their entire life just because they have an implanted device. Don't be afraid to ask your doctor to make it pretty.

12.6   Home pacemaker monitoring

Technology has provided huge advances to the pacemaker-monitoring approach. Until recently, to determine how a pace-maker was working, a specialist doctor or vendor representative in the office had to interrogate the device with a special pro-grammer, a proprietary computer that talks with the pacemak-ers through radio waves delivered by a wand.

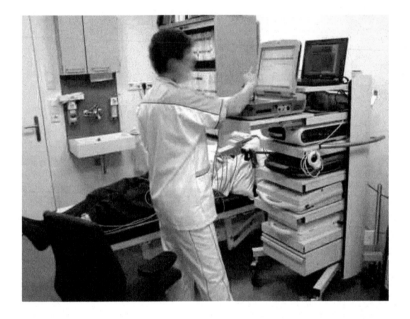

Figure 12.15: Office follow-up requires a rack of programmers to interrogate and program the various devices (With permission Jansen Medicars, medi-cars.com).

   To this day, this still remains the standard for device man-agement, thus explaining why my office is so cluttered. These programmers allow routine device evaluation, from battery life to complex adjustments of sophisticated features. How-ever, with the advent of remote technologies, much of this can now be done from your home. All the pacemaker companies now provide devices with wireless technology, with a radio fre-quency transmitter built into the header of the device can. By the way, when you get a pacemaker, be sure to ask about this feature because some hospitals restrict its use to save money.

After you go home from your pacemaker surgery, you will be provided a remote transmitter that hooks up to your phone, either a land line or cell phone. This bedside device then monitors your pacemaker and notifies the physician if something breaks. Instead of an office visit every 3 months, you can now schedule a telephone check-up, saving the commute (and making the interaction with your doctor even less personal).

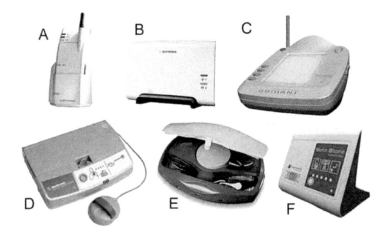

Figure 12.16: Examples of at-home remote device monitoring equipment provided by the device manufacturers (With permission, Medtronic, St. Jude, Boston Scientific, and Biotronik).

These newer wireless devices are much more sophisticated than the old telephone pacemaker checks. In fact, the technology is available to do everything now done in the physician's office remotely. The liability of reprogramming your pacemaker from afar has not been resolved, so some of these features are still on hold (this is why I encouraged my son to go to law school!).

In 2013, the TV show *Homeland* had a frightening episode where the fictional vice president was killed when someone activated his implantable cardioverter defibrillator (ICD) to induce a life-threatening arrhythmia (instead of it's normal function to end ventricular fibrillation). Of course, this is Hollywood, or is it? A real vice president, Dick Cheney, received an ICD in 2001. Cheney and his Secret Service detail anticipated this scenario depicted in *Homeland* by several years asking physicians in 2007 to deactivate his defibrillator's remote monitoring capability. Of course, with his heart transplant, Cheney no longer has an ICD.

Should you worry about someone hacking your device? Probably not—now isn't that reassuring? Theoretically, the cyber technology exists today to potentially turn a pacemaker off, or worse, make it pace so fast a life-threatening arrhythmia could be induced. Fortunately, there have been no confirmed reports of cyber criminals gaining access to a medical device and harming a patient. Relax, terrorists have found much easier ways to kill us.

12.7   Wrap: Choosing a pacemaker doctor

When choosing a pacemaker doctor, you want to keep in mind a few key points.

Device implantation, like much surgery, is best done by someone who does a lot of them. Forget the credentials and find out how often your doctor performs device implants. While EPs are generally a better choice to do your pacemaker than a general cardiologist, volume trumps credentials.

If your doctor does cardiac catheterizations, office work, or ablations most of the time, move on. However, if the doctor does at least 100 device implants a year, that is your guy or gal. Volume translates to quality, almost guaranteed. This level of experience strongly predicts that this physician has seen unusual findings and can safely get you out of trouble.

I was recently referred a patient whose doctor spent more than 4 hours trying to insert her pacemaker without success. This older doctor does only about 10 to 20 pacemakers a year and didn't promptly recognize a rare congenital ("born with") problem this lady had. This uncommon congenital abnormality, called persistent left superior vena cava, is only observed in about 3 in 1,000 people. Fortunately, this is one of those congenital problems that generally causes no harm. I recognized the issue and implanted her pacemaker successfully. Experience matters.

As someone famous once said, "Good judgment comes from experience, and experience comes from bad judgment." You want the person doing your pacemaker to have learned through bad judgment on someone else.[6]

[6] "The doctor must have put in my pacemaker wrong. Every time my husband kisses me, the garage door goes up."

13
Devices 2: So you need a defibrillator

In 2001, while Dick Cheney was vice president under George W. Bush, he had another heart attack.

He was treated with balloon angioplasty and a stent at George Washington University Hospital in D.C. Back then, knowing that interventional cardiologists often ignored rhythm issues, I sent the vice president a personal letter. In it, I outlined the findings of the MADIT study and recommended that he be proactive with his cardiologists.

If his ejection fraction (EF) was 35% or less, I suggested he probably needed an implantable cardioverter defibrillator (ICD). The MADIT study results showed a 54% greater chance of living with an ICD compared to conventional drug therapy. I received a nice form letter, likely written by an aide, thanking me for my concern.

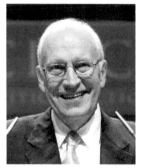

Next, as threatened in the first letter, I sent a copy of my letter to his wife, Lynne. Not 4 weeks later, Mr. Cheney received his first ICD. I like to believe it was my letter. To this day, I use the same tactic encouraging wives to convince their husbands to receive proper medical care.

Figure 13.1: Former Vice President of the United States Dick Cheney at CPAC 2011 (Photo by Gage Skidmore/Wikimedia).

Regardless of what you think of the former vice president's politics, his survival is a real testimony to modern cardiology. Here is a summary of his major cardiac issues:

- **1978:** First of five heart attacks, beginning at age 37

- **1988:** Quadruple bypass surgery after his third heart attack

- **2001:** At least his eighth cardiac catheritization and stent

- **2001:** His first ICD

- **2007:** ICD upgraded to biventricular device (with WiFi feature disabled)

- **2010:** Artificial heart pump inserted called a left ventricular assist device (LVAD)

- **2012:** Has a heart transplant that removes his old heart, stents, ICD, and leads

Cheney remains active still at age 75 and is a real "bionic" man. His story highlights the amazing success of the implantable defibrillator. ICD recipients show a greater than 50% improvement in survival rate compared to those on drug therapies alone.

13.1   History of the ICD

How the implantable defibrillator was invented is truly incredible. To escape the Nazis, Mieczyslaw "Michel" Mirowski fled Poland in 1939 to Russia and then France for his medical training. He would be the only one in his family to survive World War II.

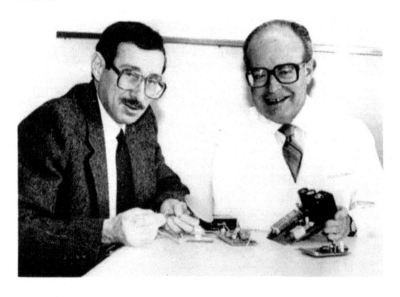

Figure 13.2: Doctors Morton Mower (left) and Michel Mirowski (right) with their first prototype of an automatic defibrillator (Photo by Ariella Rosengard, MD).

In 1961, Dr. Mirowski completed his cardiology training and returned to Israel where he became the sole cardiologist at a hospital outside Tel Aviv. In 1966, his close friend, mentor, and head of his department, Professor Harry Heller, developed a dangerous heart rhythm disorder, ventricular tachycardia (VT). Refusing hospitalization (little treatment was available at the time), Dr. Heller died suddenly just 2 weeks later at dinner with his family. This event became a major turning point in Dr. Mirowski's career.

Wondering what could have been done to prevent his mentor's death, Mirowski suggested that perhaps an external defibrillator could be miniaturized and implanted in humans. Colleagues told him that this idea was ludicrous because external defibrillators weighed 30 to 40 pounds at the time. Mirowski was not dismayed but realized that he could not pursue his research at his small Israeli hospital. He moved to the United States solely to pursue the ICD. Today, Israel is ironically a hotbed of research for American biomedical companies due to an environment more friendly to medical entrepreneurship than we presently have in the United States.

Mirowski took a job at Sinai Hospital of Baltimore, an affiliate of John Hopkins University, with the understanding that he could spend half of his time working on his idea. In 1969, Dr. Mirowski met Dr. Morton "Morty" Mower, a Hopkins-trained cardiologist. Many have described Morty as the brains, perhaps more kindly, the tinkerer, and Michel as the showman.

Regardless, these two physicians along with others developed an implantable defibrillator that they first called the "AID" for automatic implantable defibrillator, thinking of it as an aid to heart patients.

There were two problems with that name. Those of us who implant the device recognized that we actually do *something* and to say it is *automatically implanted* belittles that work.[1] More importantly, the disease AIDS came along in the 1970s and the name alone frightened many. The name was changed to the AICD for automatic implantable cardioverter defibrillator. More recently, as one company trademarked the name AICD, the most common usage is now just ICD.

Doctors Mirowski and Mower met stiff opposition to the idea of an ICD. The original manuscript was rejected from the *New England Journal of Medicine* because the reviewer stated he was "impressed but also frightened by the proposal." Two more

[1] It's not always about me, but I like to think that it is.

years passed before it was accepted in a general medical journal in 1972.

No early opposition was greater than that from the inventor of the external defibrillator and a recognized authority, Harvard cardiologist Dr. Bernard Lown, whom I described previously. In one of the most haunting medical publication mistakes, Dr. Lown and a colleague wrote an editorial in *Circulation*, the American Heart Association's (AHA) official publication, extremely critical of the ICD:[2]

> There is serious question whether an indication can be spelled out for the use of an implanted standby defibrillator ... the implanted defibrillator system represents an imperfect solution in search of a plausible and practical application ... "It was developed because it was possible."

Dr. Lown was very influential. When Drs. Mirowski and Mower presented a lecture to the annual AHA meeting showing a video of a research animal with an implanted ICD successfully shocked out of life-threatening VF, they were asked to prove that the dog hadn't been taught to play dead and wake up. Undaunted, they returned with a simultaneous EKG strip of the animal showing the VF corrected by the ICD.

Despite a lack of financial backing or grants, in 1980, Dr. Levi Watkins along with Morowski and Mower implanted the first ICD at Johns Hopkins Hospital. Dr. Roger Winkle of Stanford referred the first patient and both patient and doctor flew commercially together from San Francisco to Baltimore for the pioneering surgery. The original device required open heart surgery and was approved only for patients who had successfully survived two cardiac arrests. Fortunately, a third did not occur on the plane flight out. Without an ICD, the survival rate for a cardiac arrest is less than 10% and to survive two, less than 1%. In those early days, patients who qualified for an ICD must have had an angel on their shoulder.[3]

In 1985, shortly after arriving in San Diego, I identified a patient who had survived two cardiac arrests. Medications were ineffective then, as they are now, for cardiac arrest. I referred my patient to Stanford University Hospital, the only site in the Western United States that had the still-investigational ICD. At the time, the device weighed more than 200 grams and was implanted in a large pocket in the abdomen with open heart

[2] Lown, Bernard and Axelrod, Paul. "Implanted standby defibrillation." *Circulation*, 46:637, 1972.

[3] One of my old partners used to explain to patients who had an ICD, "With this, it will be hard to kill you unless you are shot by a jealous lover." That worked great until one guy pulled up his shirt at his first post-op visit, showed his abdominal scar, and said "Too late doc, that's already happened."

surgery to secure patch-like electrodes sewn on the outside surface of the heart. Finally, after weeks in the hospital awaiting arrival of the rare devices, my patient received an implant. He survived and returned home subsequently receiving appropriate life-saving therapy from his ICD. This advance extended his life for more than 5 years.

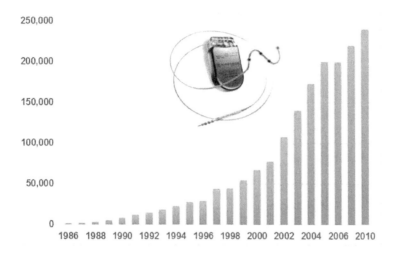

Figure 13.3: Growth of worldwide ICD implants to 250,000 annually from 1986 through 2010 (Modified from data of L Biegelsen, Wells Fargo Securities).

In 1986, the Centers for Medicare & Medicaid Services (CMS) approved the ICD for selected patients initially as a "treatment of last resort," not only requiring a prior cardiac arrest, but ICDs were also deemed unsuitable for cardiac surgery or medication therapy. Today, we know that coronary bypass surgery or medications do not prevent sudden death.

Personally, I attribute the determination of Drs. Mirowski and Mower as analogous to that of Galileo who in 1633 faced the Roman Catholic Inquisition for proposing that the earth revolved around the sun. As you will see, many more than 1 million ICDs have now been inserted in humans, saving at least 100,000 lives. The world thanks you, Michel and Morty.

13.2   ICD advances

As mentioned, the early ICDs were huge—more than 170 cc in volume and up to 280 grams (2/3 of a pound) in weight. Contrast that with today's Nanostim™ leadless pacemaker that is 1 cc and 2 grams! Imagine having something about the size of an iPad (narrower but thicker) implanted in your abdomen. And yes, I said an iPad, not an iPhone! Those first patients and doctors were pioneers.

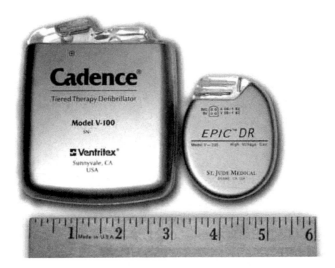

Figure 13.4: An early generation Ventritex ICD was more than 4 times the size of today's modern ICDs (With permission, St. Jude Medical).

Fortunately, advances in technology miniaturization proceeded rapidly after the clinical value of the ICD was understood. The figure shown illustrates one manufacturer's progression, though they conveniently leave out the earliest even larger devices. Today's smallest ICDs are actually about 26 cc now, one-tenth the size of the originals, with improvements continuing annually. Traditional pacemakers are less than 10 cc today.

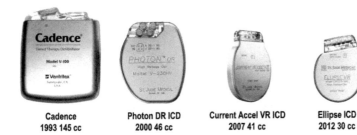

Cadence
1993 145 cc

Photon DR ICD
2000 46 cc

Current Accel VR ICD
2007 41 cc

Ellipse ICD
2012 30 cc

Figure 13.5: Examples of St. Jude Medical implantable defibrillators 1993-2012 (With permission, St. Jude Medical).

Besides making them smaller, ICDs have advanced in other

amazing ways since Mirowski and Mower's first devices. The
original devices were called "shock boxes" for good reason because they just shocked the heart when the sensed heart rate
exceeded a predetermined number. In those early years you
even had to order the device rate cut-off from the manufacturer, such as 180 bpm because nothing was adjustable, and not
uncommonly, a different rate was subsequently needed.

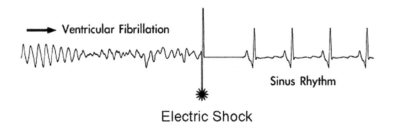

Figure 13.6: An EKG of life-
threatening VF terminated
by an ICD electric shock
back to normal sinus
rhythm (With permission,
Csaba Urban, Medical Tech
Blog).

13.3   Therapy advances

ICDs today are called that not just to distinguish them from
AIDS but because they cardiovert.[4] A much cooler advance
is anti-tachycardia pacing, astonishingly called ATP. ATP is a
way to painlessly terminate many life-threatening arrhythmias,
typically sustained VT, using a fancy pacing maneuver. As
shown, this *burst* pacing can be miraculous.

[4] Cardiovert is the term for delivering a timed shock synchronized to the rapid heartbeat to minimize risk.

   I tell patients that an ICD is like a built-in ambulance only
with the paramedic never taking a bathroom break. When the
device recognizes the heart is racing, it first determines how
bad it is. If it is sort of bad, say a rate of 170 bpm, you typically
have 15 to 30 seconds before you get dizzy or pass out. The
device promptly recognizes this and delivers ATP, or a fast
pacing pulse of around 6 to 12 beats to quickly *overdrive pace*
the VT back into normal sinus rhythm. It is a beautiful thing.
Many patients are even unaware that this brush with death has
occurred until they come in for a routine device check weeks or
months later. By the way, your ICD saved your life recently. So,
what's for lunch?

   Today, ICD devices are smart enough to recognize whether
silent ATP pacing is likely to work, and if not, such as when

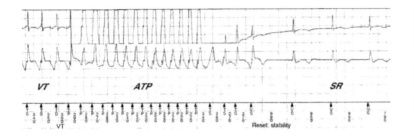

Figure 13.7: Example of VT at about 175 bpm pace-terminated by a defibrillator delivering ATP and returning the heart rhythm to normal sinus rhythm (With permission, Medtronic).

the rate is more than 220 (though all these numbers are now programmable), the device directly delivers a prompt shock within that 15-second window.

This also works terminating even more lethal arrhythmias such as VF. Of course, imagine the surprise you would feel when driving on the freeway and receiving an unexpected shock, which some colorful patients have stated "feels like a horse kicked me in the chest." Fortunately, this is quite rare and certainly beats the alternative. Over the years, I can recall only two patients who were successfully shocked and crashed their vehicle (one was a motorcycle), yet I have had hundreds who got shocks or ATP driving and did just fine. Most states allow ICD patients to drive if their device demonstrates they have not had recent or frequent shocks.

13.4   *Transvenous leads*

Even more than miniaturization, the greatest advance in ICDs has been the transvenous lead. This allows for the procedure to be safely done under x-ray guidance without opening the chest to sew on the shocking and pacing leads. There might be some dispute about which is the largest advance, but consider this: if you had your choice, would you rather have an iPad placed in your belly or your breast bone broken to get it in? Fortunately, neither option is required today.

Currently, the atrial and left-ventricular leads for an ICD are identical to those for a pacemaker. Similar to pacemakers, the mix in the United States is less than 10% single-lead ICDs, 40% dual-lead, and 50% triple-lead or cardiac resynchronization therapy ICDs, also called CRTs.

By the time we get to dual-chamber defibrillators, they are essentially just like a pacemaker, what Dick Cheney called a "pacemaker plus." All the advances of a dual-chamber pacemaker (A then V) are now in a dual-chamber ICD, plus the added benefit of treating these dangerous fast rhythms. At Scripps in 1997, I was fortunate to be the first person in the world to implant a dual-chamber ICD (and a few since then too).

The very first defibrillators required open heart surgery because the defibrillator leads looked like fly swatters, a piece of screened mesh about 2.5 x 3.5 inches with a wire that plugged into the ICD. It required two patches because the shock required electricity to travel from one patch to another.

In the early days of ICDs, only a few hospitals offered this technology, including Scripps.

When implantable ICDs were new, a patient of mine developed shortness of breath while on vacation in Las Vegas. In the ER there, he got a chest x-ray. It showed his heart surrounded by patches and wires connected to a box in his belly. In all seriousness, the ER doctor looked at it and told him, "I don't know where you have been but *don't go back there*, someone is torturing you!" When you think about it, the ER doc might have been right.

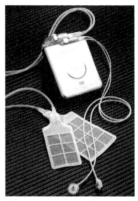

Figure 13.8: An early ICD with epicardial patches (With permission, Guidant/Boston Scientific).

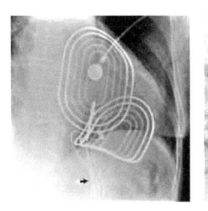 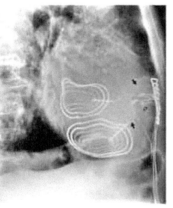

Figure 13.9: A chest x-ray showing two epicardial defibrillation patches on the heart.

It only took some genius about 15 years to realize that if you coiled a patch, it could be placed along a pacing lead and, once again, the open heart surgeons were out of work. Thus,

today, the typical ICD lead is just slightly larger than a pacemaker lead, about 1/10th of an inch in diameter. It contains
tiny wires that attach one or two shocking coils as well as pacing electrodes and a mechanism (tiny screw) to secure the lead
to the heart. The only difference between an ICD and a pacemaker's leads is this transvenous right ventricular lead (and
about $6,500).

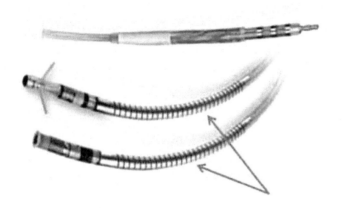

Figure 13.10: Portions of
ICD leads. The top is the
connector pin that goes
into the device header.
The middle shocking
electrode has a tined end,
and the lower lead has an
extendable and retractable
screw to affix in the right
ventricle. The arrows
show the shocking coils.
(With permission, St. Jude
Medical).

13.5   The MADIT studies

Dr. Mirowski's original colleague was Dr. Arthur Moss of the
University of Rochester, my friend and mentor from medical
school in 1975 to 1979.

Dr. Moss is an incredible scientist who devised a series of
ground-breaking clinical trials evaluating the ICD's efficacy.
The first trial was called MADIT for Multicenter Automatic
Defibrillator Implantation Trial.

Instead of limiting ICDs to patients who had survived a
cardiac arrest, this study randomly assigned patients to receive
open heart surgery for an ICD vs. a control group that received
conventional treatment, which at the time was anti-arrhythmic
medication therapy. Research subjects were defined to be at risk
for their first cardiac arrest if they had:

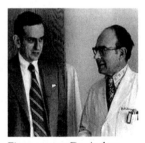

Figure 13.11: Dr. Arthur
Moss (left) with Dr. Michel
Mirowski circa 1970 (Photo
courtesy Heart Rhythm
Society Archives).

• Prior myocardial infarction (heart attack)

- EF of 35% or less

- Non-sustained VT

- Inducible arrhythmia (VT or VF) at electrophysiology (EP) study

The MADIT study results were one of the most amazing research results ever reported in the scientific literature.

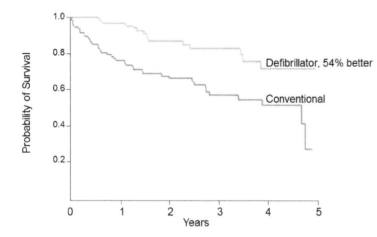

Figure 13.12: The first MADIT study results (With permission, *The New England Journal of Medicine*).

The results showed an amazing 54% greater chance of living if you were selected to have received an ICD over conventional drug therapy. Published in 1996, this study has been called "the most important clinical research of the decade."

Defibrillators were now encouraged to prevent cardiac arrest in high-risk individuals and therapy acceptance began on an exponential growth curve.

After Dr. Mirowski died, Dr. Mower went on to invent other life-saving products, including the biventricular pacemaker and defibrillator, a major advance in heart failure treatment. Similarly, Dr. Moss extended MADIT into a franchise. MADIT II found a 31% greater chance of living if an ICD was implanted in all patients with:

- Prior myocardial infarction

- EF less than or equal to 30%

- That's it! No documentation of VT or EP study needed anymore

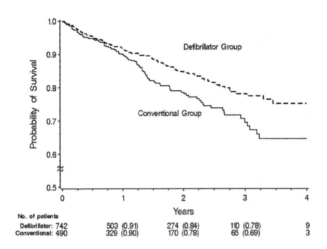

Figure 13.13: A graph from the original MADIT II publication. Note the survival difference between those who received an ICD and those treated with what was thought to be the best "conventional" therapy at the time. (With permission, *The New England Journal of Medicine*).

In 2009, 8 years after MADIT II, Dr. Moss looked back at the long-term results. The initial improvement in survival remained dramatic, finding a 37% better chance of living with the ICD in this patient group even after 8 years. In fact, those who were the healthiest, with a higher EF and less severe heart failure, did the best of all because they had no other reasons to fall ill.[5]

Economists, recognizing that we do not have infinite medical resources, have devised an economic indicator: cost per life-year saved. Money spent on premature infants is a large amount, but babies that live go on to take advantage of 70 or 80 more years of health. Alternatively, an elderly patient dying of kidney failure might not see his life prolonged much from the expense of kidney dialysis. Despite its cost, the ICD is so helpful in prolonging lives that the cost per life-year saved makes it worthwhile. Despite costing an insurer about $30,000 for surgery, the ICD is more cost effective than many other accepted medical treatments.

Even though expensive, the ICD has been proven to be highly cost effective in saving more lives than many accepted therapies. The ICD is now approved by all insurance carriers.

[5] Halfway through MADIT II, the transvenous ICD was FDA approved so you could get your ICD via a vein rather than open heart surgery, further reducing the surgical risk in the ICD group. With current transvenous systems, the MADIT II results would be even better if done today. Of course, it would be malpractice now to deny an ICD to this high-risk group today.

Neonatal ICU	$5,500
CABG x 3	$7,200
ICD conventional	$17,400
ICD MADIT	$22,800
CABG x 1	$44,200
TB skin testing	$53,100
Hemodialysis	$59,500

Table 13.1: An estimate of the cost per life-year saved for various medical therapies. Compared to some commonly accepted treatments, the ICD is cost-effective. (Adapted from Kupperman et al., "An analysis of the cost-effectiveness of the implantable defibrillator." *Circulation*, 1990;81:91-100).

It remains high on the list as one of the most successful medical advances of all time, comparable to the polio vaccine or penicillin for pneumonia.

13.6   *15 minutes of fame*

In 2001, I was getting ready to go to Orlando to the American College of Cardiology meeting where Dr. Moss was to first present the MADIT II data. Apparently because I implanted ICDs and Dr. Moss didn't, I got a call from *NBC Nightly News* with Tom Brokaw.

I needed to arrange a patient immediately for the interview. Fortuitously, I had one coming to the office who had just had a successful ICD shock.

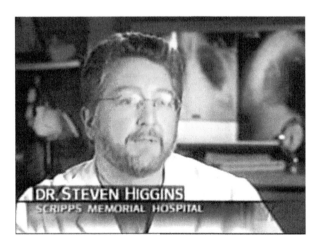

Figure 13.14: The author discussing MADIT II and its implications on *NBC Nightly News*, March 2001.

The NBC chief science and health correspondent, Robert Bazell, conducted the interview from New York with me still in La Jolla. Yet through the miracles of editing, it looked like we were in the same room. It turned out so professionally that I've probably shown it at more than 100 lectures since then.[6]

I am a bit biased about the MADIT studies as I proudly served on the executive committees for all three: MADIT, MADIT II, and MADIT-CRT along with Dr. Moss and some other EP physician leaders.

Of course, there have been other valuable clinical trials with fun names like COMPANION, DEFINITE, CABG-Patch, DINAMIT, MUSTT, and CASH among others. Despite my bias, the facts speak for themselves; MADIT remains a landmark research trial, the first to establish that many lives are saved with an implantable defibrillator. Again, we should extend our appreciation to Morty, Michel, and Art.

13.7   Reasons for an ICD

As noted, the ICD is now approved in the United States and elsewhere for preventing sudden death in high-risk individuals. The criteria are divided into secondary reasons (already had a life-threatening arrhythmia) and primary prevention (at risk but no sudden death yet). Today, the approved indications (reason for doing it) for an ICD are fairly simple:

- After any survived cardiac arrest without reversible cause (secondary prevention)

- Any patient with an EF of less than or equal to 40% and prior heart attack at least 40 days ago

- Any patient with an EF of less than or equal to 35% without prior heart attack (nonischemic cardiomyopathy)

Of course, the ICD is not for everyone in these summarized groups. A reversible cause for cardiac arrest includes an acute myocardial infarction (heart attack), ingestion of toxins, and so on. Common sense requires that patients also be excluded if they have a limited prognosis from other illness (less than 1 year to live), a recent heart attack, coronary intervention, or bypass surgery (because sometimes left ventricular function improves during the next 90 days). Today, patients who are waiting after a coronary event to see if they remain at-risk for sudden death go home with a ZOLL LifeVest®. The LifeVest is

[6] If you Google "Steve Higgins," the announcer from Jimmy Fallon's *Tonight Show* might appear first. He seems to be more famous than me despite having little skill at cardiology. He must also have seen my *NBC News* video because he sent me a funny e-mail about it. Interestingly, I never have trouble getting a dinner reservation in New York.

a high-fashion wearable external defibrillator that patients must parade around in for up to 90 days while awaiting insurance OK for an ICD.

13.8 A typical ICD surgery experience

How exactly is ICD surgery done today?

If you meet the criteria outlined above, the surgery is often elective because findings, such as a weak heart with a low EF, are most commonly uncovered by a routine outpatient echocardiogram (ultrasound study). You will be instructed to arrive with an empty stomach 2 hours early to get an IV, lab work, and the all-important wallet biopsy (also called insurance verification).

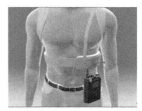

Figure 13.15: The ZOLL LifeVest® provides long-term external defibrillation while awaiting insurance approval for the implanted version. I always tell my LifeVest patients to take a really quick shower when they take it off (With permission, ZOLL).

Figure 13.16: The wallet biopsy (With artist's permission).

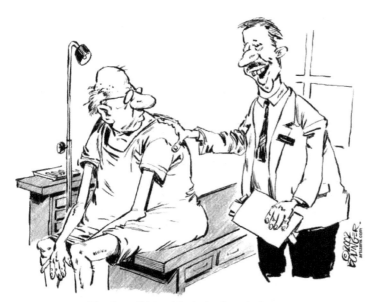

"Fred, we'll be able to better design your treatment plan right after your wallet biopsy."

You will then be transported to an EP lab, which resembles a typical operating room. The only difference is that the doctors are more handsome and there are loads of computer monitors and wires.

An anesthesiologist makes sure that you are comfortably asleep, assures that you won't have pain (other than for the

IV), and you will likely not remember your surgery experience at all. In addition to general anesthesia, a local anesthetic is applied at the site so it remains numb for a few hours even after you awaken.

A device implant is relatively minor compared to open heart surgery.[7] An incision is made of about 1.5 to 2 inches, typically either in the fold just below your shoulder, or if you want the scar to be hidden, in the lateral chest near the armpit or next to the breast (for women or big-chested men). The huge advance over open heart surgery is to place the lead transvenously (which means, "through a vein"—rule number one once again).

[7] Do you know the definition of minor surgery? Surgery on someone else.

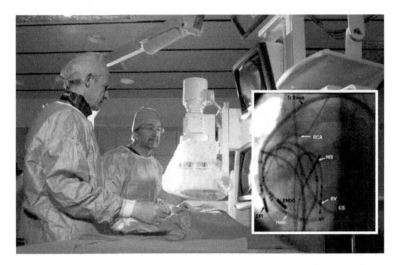

Figure 13.17: A handsome EP doc and an assistant in an EP lab mapping and placing ablation catheters with x-ray imaging.

Access to the heart is achieved by inserting a small needle in a vein in the upper chest and then advancing a wire followed by a peel-away sheath (hollow tube, like a straw) to maintain access. The lead is like a large piece of cooked spaghetti that is threaded into the vein through the sheath. It is stiffened temporarily by inserting a tiny wire into the middle that allows it to be advanced into the heart under x-ray (fluoroscopy) guidance. The wire or stylet is removed after the lead is properly positioned.

The leads are secured with either tines (plastic barbs) that later scar into the heart or, more commonly today, tiny screws. After the leads are positioned correctly on x-ray, they are sutured down so that they won't move. Then, the device, in this case an ICD, is connected to the leads with more tiny screws that secure the pins to the device header.

One of the most difficult parts of the surgery is to remember, righty tighty, lefty loosy, or is it righty loosy? The defibrillator generator, also called the can or battery, is next placed in a surgical pocket under the skin. Creating this pocket is what requires anesthesia.

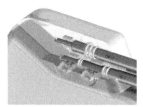

Figure 13.18: View of an ICD header with electrodes attached, set screws not shown (With permission, Biotronik).

Because most ICDs are quite small today and many Americans quite large, these pockets are commonly created in the soft tissue (a nice word for fat) above the muscle of your upper chest. Because a typical ICD is only 1/2 inch thick, it doesn't protrude much, usually far less than your collar bone. If you happen to be a runway model with anorexia (I know that's redundant), the defibrillator can be placed under the muscle of the chest wall to make it even less visible.

That's about it. The pocket is closed with absorbable stitches, followed by really expensive medical Super Glue (really), a Saran Wrap-like dressing attached, and the huge bill prepared. I typically send most patients home after a few hours of observation because even with our state-of-the-art new hospital, most people like sleeping in their own beds.[8]

Immediately after surgery, I instruct patients (and their families) that they are to not play golf or tennis or lift more than 10 pounds for 1 month. Also, most men beg me to tell their wives that they can't do the dishes or take out the trash. To hide my gender bias, 70% of ICDs in the United States are still in men because women get their heart disease later in life.

One of my favorite ICD stories is about a colleague's patient. This patient, who had an ICD, was walking to his car after losing most of his money at a local casino. In the parking lot, he was confronted by an armed robber who told him, "Hand over all your money!" The ICD patient said he had none and the robber said, "Don't lie to me or I will shoot." Despite the gun, the guy panicked and started running away. Just then, his defibrillator shocked him (probably from a really fast normal rate, sinus tachycardia, from the anxiety). He fell to the ground, patting himself to see if he could figure out where the bullet entered. The thief realizing he hadn't even pulled the trigger, ran off in fear, and the guy avoided both the robbery and a

[8] These days, a pacemaker costs a hospital about $5,000 and an ICD about $15,000 to $20,000, including leads. However, when you include all the other expenses, the bill is typically more than $75,000 to 100,000 for less than a 24-hour stay. Most plans pay about one-quarter of the cost. Fortunately, ICD surgery is covered by insurance, so the typical patient has an out-of-pocket expense of $2,500 or less.

possible assault. I told you that defibrillators save lives.

13.9   Twiddler's syndrome

In the never-ending verification that "no good deed goes un-punished" we must address Twiddler's syndrome. Surprisingly common, patients might actually twist their implanted device, whether a pacemaker or defibrillator and mess up the leads, often twisting them entirely out of the heart. Although this occurs in up to 5% of implants, I have never yet had a patient admit it was self-induced. Frequently, I get blamed (probably a "shoot the messenger" issue). Rarely, I have had the spouse say, "Now honey, you are always rubbing your device. In fact, you even once showed me how you had it on its edge!" Some fun guy actually named this Twiddler's syndrome, a name that has stuck for obvious reasons.

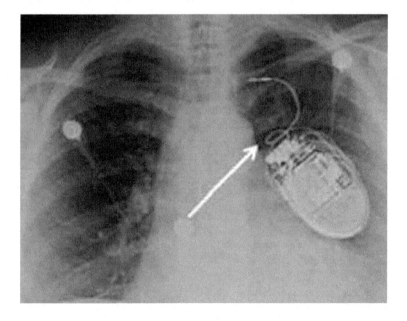

Figure 13.19: Findings in a patient with Twidder's syndrome. This generator has been flipped about 20 times, pulling the leads entirely out of the heart.

Seriously, I think Twiddler's is just a subconscious maneuver to reduce pain. As we all have experienced, pain might be diminished by rubbing, attributed to *pressure nerves* that reduce or distribute the sensation of pain by recruiting other nerves near the affected area. Others have suggested that twisting your pacemaker is just like apes who enjoy grooming themselves or humans (or apes) who feel better after a hug. I have no better explanation. All I know is that if you have enough soft tissue (read "fat") around your defibrillator, there is a chance you can actually pull the leads out of your heart by rubbing it so much that it flips around and around. My patients now get instructions to never touch the surgery site for a month because this is typically when this occurs. I also instruct spouses to watch for this flipping activity because we all know that when our spouse tells us to stop doing something we stop.

What happens when I discover a patient has twiddled his leads out of their proper locations? Well, I first show him the x-ray for educational purposes, then bring him back to surgery. The old leads are removed and new ones are inserted. Still, about 25% are repeat offenders because when you put your mind to it, you can break a 0-silk suture quite easily. If you use anything thicker than 0-silk, like zip ties, the leads will be damaged.[9] Perhaps Twiddler's patients are just ahead of the curve, anticipating the future where we will have leadless devices.

[9] Victor Parsonnet, a famous pacemaker doctor, invented a Dacron pouch to hold the device in place just for this problem, though it is no longer available.

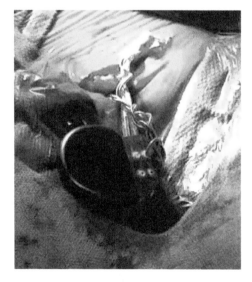

Figure 13.20: Twiddler's syndrome—the lead has been pulled back about 12 inches, barely remaining in a blood vessel. The twiddled leads, though coiled, remain attached to the generator.

13.10   Subcutaneous ICDs

One manufacturer has an FDA-approved subcutaneous ICD, the Boston Scientific EMBLEM S-ICD™. When in early development, it was called a leadless ICD but then it was discovered that it worked better with small leads that are just inserted in the soft tissue above the rib cage. It really does not have any leads within veins and thus avoids problems like Twiddler's syndrome and lead dislodgement. The current generation is relatively bulky and does not have traditional pacing capability. It truly is just a "shock box." To achieve the proper vector, the generator must be implanted on the left lateral chest wall at a location where there is not much soft tissue (or fat) often causing discomfort. It is likely that future generations will continue to get smaller.

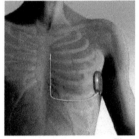

Figure 13.21: The S-ICD™ has no leads inside the chest, they reside outside the rib cage in the soft tissue of the chest wall (With permission, Boston Scientific).

Most commonly, it is implanted in patients who only need a shock box. For example, I had a teenage swimmer who had a cardiac arrest in a pool. By the way, if you schedule your cardiac arrest, don't do it while swimming. Fortunately, he recovered without permanent brain injury from the near-drowning. Anyway, he is young and still growing, so a device without intravascular leads was preferable. For the future, if the device size can be substantially improved and a painless pacing achieved from this configuration, the subcutaneous ICD could become the standard.

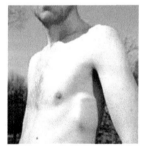

Figure 13.22: The generator and leads might remain evident in thin patients (With permission, Boston Scientific).

13.11   ICD shocks

So, now you have an ICD. What happens if the damn thing goes off?

Fortunately, this is actually relatively rare, with about two-thirds never receiving a shock their entire life. Like other preventive medicine, not everyone who gets an ICD will ever be treated, but we can't reliably predict who will benefit.

The most common treatment from an ICD is that painless treatment called anti-tachycardia pacing (ATP) that I mentioned earlier. If you develop a relatively stable heart racing, your ICD will actually deliver really fast silent pacing pulses, for no more than a few seconds, in an attempt to stop it. That works up to 90% of the time in slower VTs (the slower the better, but it works best below 180 bpm). Patients are typically unaware that the device saved their lives.[10]

Of course, ICD shocks do happen, and usually when you least expect it. One of my very first patients had his first shock while having sex. Another of my very early patients had his first shock while mowing the lawn. His neighbor watched him collapse, awaken, look around, and then sheepishly finish mowing. Of course, the neighbor never offered to help. The patient realized that if he called an ambulance the lawn would remain half mowed. So he finished and then called paramedics. Today, I would encourage him not to call 911 at all; he could finish mowing the lawn. As amazing as it sounds, an appropriate ICD shock is often an isolated event, over before you even figure out what happened. If you have just one, it is usually fine to just carry on. Of course, you should make an appointment to see your EP doctor who will interrogate the device to see why it fired. Showing a person how his or her life was saved is another job perk. Did I thank Morty and Michel enough yet?

13.12   Post-op issues

As mentioned, ICD surgery is fairly minor these days with many patients going home the same day as the implant procedure. I mentioned the need for limiting left arm motion until the leads scar into the heart, usually safe after a month. Of course after the section above, you will never be a twiddler, will you? It is also important to avoid driving until you are well and haven't received a recent shock, though often that is safe within the first week or two. The infection risk is the same as that with pacemakers, not prevented with antibiotics and far more common after a generator change than a new implant.

Office follow-up is usually 1 to 2 weeks post-op to check the wound, remove the dressing, and re-explain what happened because many don't really remember. A 2003 study from Britain found that up to 80% of patients don't remember what their doctor talked about in the office visit (likely higher when patients are just waking up from anesthesia). For this reason, I like to write down instructions and provide pictures as reminders. Plus, having a picture as a memento makes that $100,000 bill a little more palatable (not really).

[10] One of the most enjoyable parts of my job is to show patients how their ICD saved their life (the rhythm is recorded in the device and can be printed) when they come in for a routine office visit. See, I told you that surgery you didn't want was worth it. Every day forward is a gift, make the most of it.

13.13   *Wrap*

We owe a huge debt of gratitude to the pioneers who invented an implantable way to shock your heart, an idea that once must have sounded way out there. Here are a few defibrillator takeaways:

- The ICD is one of medicine's most amazing advances.

- The studies are clear, if you have a weak heart (EF less than or equal to 35%), get an ICD, period.

- If you have an ICD, you are lucky to be alive today because the early patients went through hell to get a defibrillator.

- If you get an ICD, don't "twiddle" it.

14
Ablation

The term ablation comes from the Latin word "ablat" meaning "taken away" or "removed." Cardiac ablation is a procedure that is used to scar or wall-off small areas in your heart that might be causing heart rhythm issues. The surgery is performed using a catheter guided into the blood vessels and on into the heart.

It is still debated about who did the very first human catheter ablation, either Mel Scheinman at UC San Francisco or Geoffrey Hartzler in Kansas City (who also did one of the first angioplasties, a real cowboy apparently).

Just last month, I attended a lecture by Dr. Mel Scheinman, still brilliant at age 80 and still at UC San Francisco doing electrophysiology (EP), where he has been since 1967. He gave several pearls of wisdom for EP doctors to remember:

- Don't keep doing the wrong thing again and again and expect a different result.

- If you burn enough to see white smoke, move on; you are not electing a pope.

- When people faint, dehydration suddenly becomes an epidemic (a commonly overused excuse, often ignoring a potentially serious undiagnosed arrhythmia).

- Not all ventricular tachycardia (VT) is real, such as "V Tap."

What is "V Tap" you ask? When I was a medical resident in Colorado, we had a nice Cardiac Care Unit with a view of the Rockies. One indigent patient seemed healthy, but whenever he was about to be discharged, he had another episode of what looked like very serious VT, a rapid racing of his heart at about 200 bpm. The alarms would go off, the nurses and residents would rush in the room, but he looked fine just as his heart rhythm went back to normal. This must have happened 10 times. I got this brilliant idea to turn off the loud alarm. The next time our friend had VT, we tiptoed into his room and caught him looking at his own monitor, tapping the cables on his EKG to simulate VT. We labeled it "V Tap" and even published the case report.

14.1   How ablation works

There are two general methods for performing heart ablations:

1. Radiofrequency (RF) ablations using heat energy

2. Cryoablation using freezing cold

When ablations were first performed, there was no proven energy source to destroy abnormal heart tissue other than a surgeon's scalpel. Because we didn't want to open the chest every time, someone suggested that an external defibrillator could be focused to create energy to destroy heart tissue. Using common electrical equipment, a standard defibrillator was attached to a catheter (stiff wire with metal electrodes) and placed first in an animal and then humans to see what would happen. Actually, back then, we used to say that new treatments were first done on Europeans, then dogs, and then Americans.

In the late '80s direct current (DC) ablation was gaining traction at a few select hospitals in an attempt to cure several arrhythmias. At Scripps, I wanted to try it. I persuaded our biomedical department into making an adapter to the regular defibrillator to connect to a standard four-pole EP catheter. I paid for a plane ticket for a doctor at Cedars Sinai Medical Center in LA, Billy Mandel, to come to San Diego for the day to show me how to do it. All went well and Billy was home in time for cocktails, and I was now the local expert. This was a real example of see one, do one, teach one. Thus, the first ablation in San Diego was done at Scripps in 1986, the third center in California (Scheinman at UC-San Francisco, Mandell at Cedars, and then us). As primitive as this was, it surpassed open heart surgery in an attempt to cure a serious arrhythmia.

That worked well until someone videotaped what we were doing inside the heart. In the early '90s a room full of EP doctors watched in stunned silence as a close-up of a DC shock ablation looked just like the Hiroshima nuclear blast with a giant explosion, followed by a gas bubble and barotrauma (Latin for a bomb) to the heart tissue.

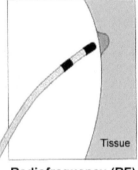
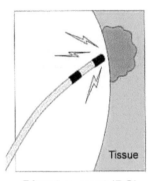

Radiofrequency (RF) energy   **Direct current (DC) energy**

Figure 14.1: RF ablation creates a much more controlled injury to heart tissue than the older DC ablation (Photo courtesy Heart Rhythm Society Archives).

The next energy source tried was called RF for *radiofrequency* energy. Compared to the explosions of DC current, RF is like a BB gun. Today, we can deliver RF energy through irrigated catheters, similar to a shower head, that keeps the tip from getting warm or forming "char" (just like on your BBQ'd ribs), thus allowing higher energies for longer times. Irrigated RF ablation delivers a controlled burn to just the heart tissue next to a catheter damaging no more than 1/4 to 1/2 of an inch of diseased heart tissue.

Over the years, many other energy sources have been tried on the heart. I was part of an early trial with microwave energy, but the patient kept spinning off the platter in the oven. Plus, it didn't even work well to keep our food warm. Lasers were also tried. I know one doctor who actually shot a hole in his shoe with a laser (like Austin Powers) testing it just before trying it on a patient.

If heat works, how about cold?

Other than RF, *cryoablation* is the only approved energy

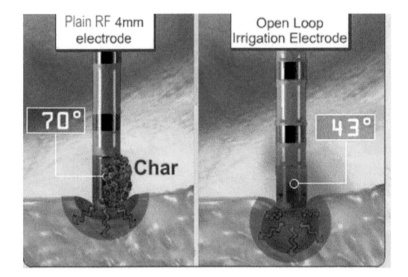

Figure 14.2: An irrigated ablation catheter bathes the tip and tissue with fluid to prevent overheating, allowing for a safer and more controlled ablation. Temperatures are in centigrade (normal body temp is 37 °C) (With permission, Biosense Webster).

source for cardiac ablation. It is presently only available for atrial fibrillation (AF) ablation, actually the hardest of all arrhythmias to treat. Cryoablation has the most potential for ablation because it can theoretically be reversed, unlike RF. If you see something wrong after delivering a lesion, like complete heart block, just stop and warm up the heart, and the tissue should recover. Back when we were doing open heart surgery ablations, we used a similar type of cryoablation, with a cool refrigerated tool that could destroy tissue and be reversed with a quick dousing from a double soy latte (actually a pitcher of sterile warm saline).

In 2009, Medtronic bought a nearby Carlsbad company, Ablation Frontiers, with a product appropriately named Arctic Front that provides catheters for cryoablation. The Arctic Front system employs a balloon that is inflated in a pulmonary vein where instant cooling destroys the tissue in a smooth circle around that vein in just one application, theoretically at least. There is a small vocal subset of EP doctors, including one of my partners, who swear by it, claiming it is better than RF.

A very useful clinical trial, cleverly named "Fire & Ice" should be published in 2017, a direct head-to-head comparison of RF vs. cryoablation for AF ablation. Until it is out, your guess is as good as mine as to which is better. For now, I save

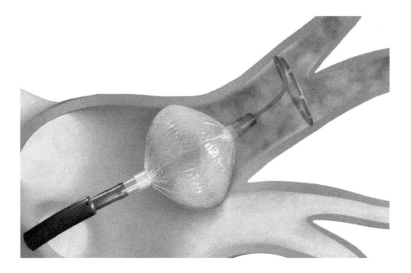

Figure 14.3: A cryoablation balloon in a pulmonary vein (With permission, Medtronic).

the ice for my Scotch and stick to RF but what do I know about predicting the future?

14.2 When is ablation needed?

There are two basic types of arrhythmias, the first depends on a wire or pathway to conduct electricity around and around in a circle, called *reentry*. The second is a focal area that takes off on its own.

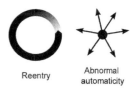

Reentry   Abnormal automaticity

Figure 14.4: Diagram illustrating the paths of the two types of arrhythmia "short circuits" in the heart: reentry and focal (abnormal autmaticity) (With permission, ECGpedia.org).

Problems like atrial flutter and common supraventricular tachycardia (SVT), called atrioventricular (AV) node reentry, are the former. They are especially amenable to ablation because all you have to do is snip the wire and you are cured. Of course, just like in the movies defusing the bomb, the stress is in trying to determine, "Do I snip the red wire or the blue wire?"

For atrial flutter, you ablate a line along a small area in the lower-right atrium, called the cavotricuspid isthmus, and it can't recirculate anymore. For SVT, you burn the *slow pathway* adjacent to the normal AV node conduction the arrhythmia will stop. Similarly, for Wolff-Parkinson-White syndrome (WPW) or for premature ventricular contractions (PVCs) or most VTs, you just map, ablate, and order lunch. With current techniques, these arrhythmias are cured with just one ablation procedure in about **95%** of patients. That beats the cure rate for almost anything in medicine.

Focal (also called automatic or ectopic) arrhythmias are those arrhythmias, such as atrial tachycardia, non-ischemic VTs, and inappropriate sinus tachycardia. They too can be cured with ablation, but the major challenge is the difficulty initiating the arrhythmia before ablating so that it can be located.

An arrhythmia that you can induce is a great marker for success when you can no longer induce it after ablation. These harder-to-reproduce focal arrhythmias thus have a lower success rate, more like **80 to 90%** cure rates.

Finally, AF is a different animal and success rates are about **60%** if doctors are honest about the long-term outcome. AF ablation is discussed in more detail in Chapter 16.

14.3   *Where ablations are performed*

There are a number of different arrhythmias that ablation can be cure. These range from easy-to-cure reentry arrhythmias like atrial flutter to harder-to-cure arrhythmias like AF.

14.3.1   *Atrial flutter*

Atrial flutter is consistently curable with a 95% success rate. Typical flutter has been proven to be due to a giant circle of electrical reentry rotating around both atria at a rate of 250 to 300 bpm.

Fortunately, the ventricles typically follow in a direct fraction of that. For example, if the atria are at 300, untreated, the ventricular rate (your pulse) will be half that, 150. This is enough to make you feel lousy but not die, which you would if your pulse actually were 300.

Because of the anatomy of the atria, it is essential that this large electrical circuit course through a small area between two electrically silent structures, the tricuspid valve and the inferior vena cava. Now, Mr. Flutter, we gotcha. Ablate in that discrete area, called the CTI for cavotricuspid isthmus. RF creates such small burns that a line of ablation lesions needs to be laid down.

After completion, we pace and confirm that the burns have created a line of block. Not uncommonly, a small area might

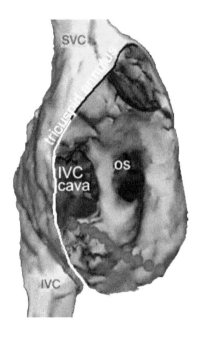

Figure 14.5: A 3D map of the inside of the right atrium. The red dots are ablation burns creating a line of block from the tricuspid valve to the inferior vena cava, the so-called CTI (Image by Wes Todd, CES).

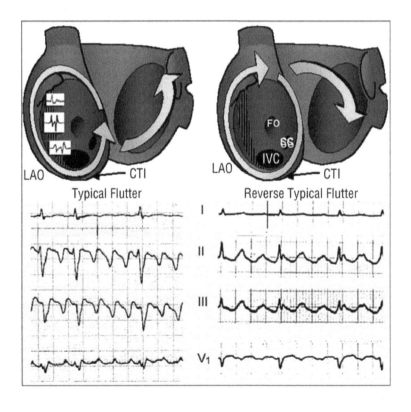

Figure 14.6: Atrial flutter from the right atrium is either typical (counter-clockwise loop) or less commonly, reverse (clockwise). Both involve conduction through the CTI and are often cured with ablation (Image by H. Tran, MD).

need to be touched up. When CTI block is created, it cures
atrial flutter 95% of the time. A colleague at UC San Diego,
Greg Feld, first figured this out. Unfortunately, not all flutters
are typical, so sometimes the success rates are less than 95%.
Also, unfortunately, even after a successful flutter ablation,
there is still about a 25% chance of later developing its sister arrhythmia, AF, at some point in your life. So, you might become
a repeat customer.

14.3.2   PSVT, SVT, and AV node reentry

Call it what you want, paroxysmal supraventricular tachycardia
(PSVT) is the most common regular arrhythmia we ablate. For
some reason, the atrioventricular (AV) node, that magical electrical structure smack dab in the middle of the heart (the soul of
the heart), frequently develops into two pathways. This division
usually doesn't happen until age 20 to 30 or older but then can
present with a sudden rapid regular racing of the heart, stuck
at a rate, such as 160 bpm. This type of reentry most commonly
involves a premature beat followed by conduction down the
slow AV node pathway turning right around and going up the
fast pathway. Unless you want to come to the ER every time
your heart races, ablation is the best treatment.

An SVT ablation involves two steps. First you need to do
what my heart surgeons call "some of that pacing crap."
Through temporary pacing catheters inserted through a vein
in the groin, we deliver carefully timed pacing impulses in the
right atrium or ventricle. This technique is used to reproduce
the clinical arrhythmia and figure out where it originates. With
AV node reentry, you usually can cause the SVT to recur and
then you can map it to make sure you have the location right. If
you can't reproduce the sustained SVT, it is common to at least
find the telltale evidence of dual pathways. Then, part two, we
kill it.

A slow pathway ablation is also called an AV node modification. The goal is to eliminate the extra pathway without
harming the normal AV node conduction. The slow pathway is
like an appendix because it has no functioning purpose. As this
pathway dies, it lets out a little scream that we call AJR, or accelerated junctional rhythm, just to let you know we are in the

correct spot. We know we are done when we see this AJR and can no longer induce the SVT. This ablation also works about 95% of the time with risks of about 1%, including that rare need for a pacemaker.

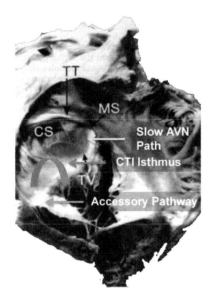

Figure 14.7: The "soul of the heart" showing how the small area between the tricuspid valve and coronary sinus is the location for many different treatable arrhythmias.

It still amazes me that this small location, just adjacent to the AV node, is where so much electrical action is in EP. Literally, in the dead center of the heart, all within a square inch of each other are the AV node, slow pathway, bundle branches, many WPW pathways, and the coronary sinus. We use the coronary sinus for access to the left ventricle for biventricular pacing, ICD permanent leads, and also for ablations to record and sometimes ablate pathways in the septum or left heart. All within an inch; no wonder we need mapping to know where we are. Because this is the "spiritual" center for all arrhythmias, I call it the soul of the heart.

Don't forget that *not* getting an ablation due to fear of a pacemaker or something else carries significant risks too. Recurrent heart racing can cause you to faint, crash your car, hit your head, or otherwise spoil your date night.

14.3.3   Wolff, Parkinson, and White syndrome (WPW)

Remember the three guys standing together for their selfie, doctors Wolff, Parkinson, and White?

WPW syndrome is the name for an electrical abnormality present from birth (though usually not showing up until teenage years or later) due to an extra wire or pathway from the atria to the ventricles. The heart is amazingly designed. Despite all this electricity to keep it running, no impulses can get from the upper chambers to the lower chambers because both AV valves, the tricuspid and mitral, are electrically silent. Thus, in a normal heart, you can only go down the AV node, which is designed to keep your heart from racing. In WPW, this extra pathway can occur anywhere along those supposedly electrically silent areas near the valves.

The most common location for WPW is along the left heart, on the side between the left atrium and ventricle. To ablate this little pathway, EP doctors need to get there, either backwards (retrograde) through the aorta, then into the left ventricle and to the mitral valve annulus.

More commonly, we just insert a sheath (hollow tube) across the septum between the right and left atria. With current tools, including echocardiograms and pressure guidance, this technique is very safe and the little hole seals over after removal. Then, you place your ablation catheter right on the accessory pathway from the atrial side of the mitral valve and fire away. Frequently, WPW disappears with just one RF burn, a beautiful thing.

Delta wave of WPW   **No delta wave; patient cured**

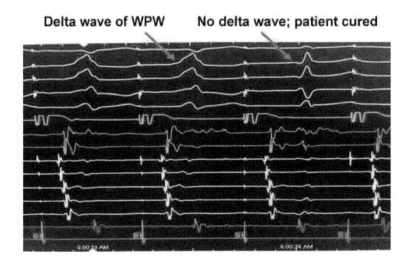

Figure 14.8: A patient's life is changed in one heartbeat. The first arrow shows the delta wave of WPW. As ablation energy is delivered, the next beat is now normal, WPW cured for life. Before the ablation, the patient had daily episodes of SVT at rates to 200 bpm.

As shown, the patient's life is changed in just one heartbeat. The delta wave showing EKG evidence of this extra pathway literally disappears for good from one beat to the next. Like politics, though (well, not that bad), things don't always go as planned. Sometimes, the pathway is actually a band of fibers, so you need to burn a larger area. Sometimes, your catheter can't just get right on the pathway, so you have to attack it from the other side (ventricular insertion). However, it usually works out great, again with a 95% chance of a permanent cure. Today, most patients go home the same day as the procedure, cured and back to work in a few days.

Sometimes, WPW presents in a *concealed* fashion, which means there is no delta wave on an EKG showing electrical conduction from A to V because it only conducts backwards, from V to A, hence concealed. Still, if it causes heart racing, the EP mantra is to kill it. Ablation is a little like when a surgeon goes duck hunting, "fire, ready, aim." [1]

Only about half of WPW syndrome pathways are located on the left heart, so before ablating it is necessary to map and confirm the location. The second most common site is in the soul of the heart again, a posteroseptal pathway just behind the AV node. Other common locations are directly in front of the node, called anteroseptal, as well as other areas in the right heart, called the right free wall. Success rates are nearly as good in these alternative locations, though, if the pathway is next to the AV node, the risk of a pacemaker surfaces again. Usually, at the time of ablation, we can determine whether the pathway is too close to the normal AV node and rarely have to stop and wake the patient up without ablating. As discussed in the arrhythmias chapter, there is a small but real risk of sudden death with untreated WPW from something bad called atrioventricular fibrillation. Thus, it is good to get WPW cured if you can. Curing WPW is really the most amazing thing we EP docs do.

[1] Three doctors were in the hospital cafeteria bragging about their dogs. The discussion got heated, so they decided to have a "dog off" contest the next weekend. The first dog, belonging to the internist, began speaking and recited all the Krebs cycle enzymes (don't worry about what that is). The surgeon took a scalpel out of his vest pocket, twirled it in the air and his dog caught it in his mouth. He then tripped the internist's dog and quickly took out his appendix. The radiologist was very impressed, admitting defeat. All his dog could do was screw the other two and take the afternoon off.

14.3.4   *Ventricular tachycardia ablation*

If we can just ablate VT and cure it, why do we need implantable cardioverter defibrillators (ICDs)?

The simple answer is that ICDs essentially always work

but ablations don't, and you don't want to fool around with sudden death. Nevertheless, there are three situations when VT ablation might be a great option:

- Normal hearts with VT caused by a short circuit most commonly in the right ventricular outflow tract

- Frequent PVCs that contribute to heart weakening and intolerable symptoms

- Weakened hearts that have VT causing too many ICD shocks

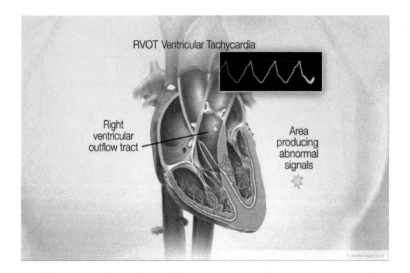

Figure 14.9: The right ventricular outflow tract is a common location for healthy hearts to develop frequent PVCs or VT that can be eliminated with catheter ablation.

Just like we don't know why AF comes from the pulmonary veins, we don't know why healthy hearts sometimes develop VT short circuits. The most common location for this to occur is in the right ventricular outflow tract, just before blood goes into the lungs. This area can be accurately mapped and this type of VT cured with up to a 95% success rate.

We all have premature ventricular contractions (PVCs), those skipped beats that come from the lower chambers, typically up to a hundred or more a day. However, when they occur very frequently, such as 10,000 of the 80,000 heart beats you have in a day, they can spell trouble. These very frequent PVCs are like bad timing in your engine that causes the pump to weaken causing fatigue, palpitations, and dizziness. With modern tools, these isolated PVCs can be mapped and ablated, decreasing but not eliminating all PVCs.

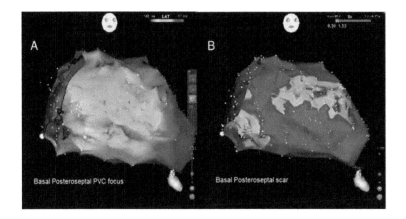

Figure 14.10: An activation map showing the origin of a PVC focus (orange). In the same view, another photo from a 3D voltage or scar map showing the area selected was diseased before the ablation, explaining the mechanism of this patient's arrhythmia.

14.3.5   AF ablation

AF ablation is discussed in detail in Chapter 16, which deals with all aspects of management for this common problem.

14.4   A typical ablation experience

Lisa is a 34-year-old nurse who has a 15-year history of arrhythmias and heart trouble. She has a very rare heart problem, called arrhythmogenic right ventricular dysplasia. Her situation is applicable regardless of whether you or your loved one is young and needs an SVT ablation (PSVT or atrial flutter), middle-aged and needs an AF ablation (called a PVI, pulmonary vein isolation), or older and needs an ischemic VT ablation.

Lisa already has an ICD and had a prior VT ablation more than 10 years ago. She showed up in the Scripps ER after getting multiple shocks for VT from her ICD that converted the VT to regular sinus rhythm with a shock saving her life. For comparison, this story could just as easily have been about another patient with SVT who required adenosine or a cardioversion in the ER, still coming to an ablation procedure.[2]

Anyway, Lisa was previously managed at another hospital that we will call Mount St. Elsewhere to protect the guilty.

[2] Remember, the answer is ablation. Now what was the question?

Despite her rare and ill-understood heart problem, her complex defibrillator, and her young age, a general cardiologist, who did some device implants at Mount St. Elsewhere, was managing her.[3]

After her shocks, Lisa spent one night in our hospital, had her medications adjusted, and was scheduled for an ablation (despite five EP labs at Scripps, it takes several weeks to get scheduled) because I knew medication wasn't a long-term solution. In fact, Lisa being a bright nurse, also knew the medicine (amiodarone) wasn't good for her long term. True to form, before her scheduled ablation, Lisa had another painful shock from her ICD for rapid VT resulting in another ER visit, this time back to Mount St. Elsewhere. As a result, I expedited Lisa's ablation to an earlier date.

I honestly tell patients that the worst part of the ablation or surgery is getting the IV in the pre-procedure area. This is generally true, not because the IV is a problem but because it is all you will remember; for the rest of your procedure you will be comfortably under anesthesia.

After her IV, Lisa was transported by our beautiful and experienced staff into one of our EP labs.[4]

The anesthesiologist administered IV medications, which commonly includes the drug, propofol. Her vital signs were skillfully monitored, including blood pressure, heart rate, pulse oximetry, BIS brain monitor, and temperature through an esophageal probe (more accurate and also lets us know if the esophagus is getting hot from ablation burning).

Only after she was comfortably asleep did the real work start. Lisa was prepped and draped. For long cases like hers, a Foley catheter was inserted into her bladder. Where the EP catheters were inserted, Lisa was shaved and was now "prepped" with sterile soap solution followed by sterile cover sheets. We used the groin area on the right side because the blood vessels (femoral vein and artery) are large and because I am right handed and it is easier. "All roads lead to Rome," so any large vein can be used to insert a catheter back to the heart.

At this point, I stopped playing on the computer and got to work. For Lisa, I inserted four sheaths or large flexible tubes into the femoral blood vessels.

Numbing medicine was first applied (the area remained

[3] In fact, he had recently completed a generator change for Lisa, which incidentally I was disappointed to find left this pretty 34-year-old with a large stretching scar on her upper chest so she could not wear many attractive clothes. Don't be afraid to ask your doctor to "make it pretty."

[4] I must mention again that volume in a program (number of cases), and volume of procedures your doctor has performed, is probably the single biggest predictor of a successful outcome. Insist that your procedure be done by someone who does a lot of them every month. Don't go somewhere where EP is a part-time specialty. At Scripps, we have five full-time EP labs, two more in the development stages, and 14 EP doctors. Equally important, the trained EP staff have seen all the routine and all the challenging cases, so they are comfortable in what to do in case something happens. Avoiding trouble and getting out of it are important skills you want your team to have that come only from experience.

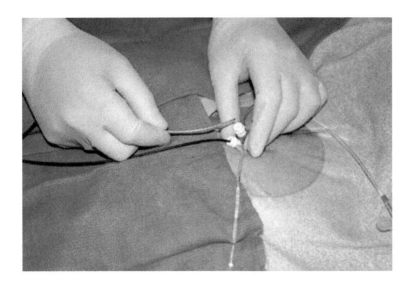

Figure 14.11: Ablation catheters entering sheaths in the groin vessels.

numb for a few hours after Lisa woke up) and then a small hollow needle was used to access the vessel, followed by a small wire inserted through the needle. The needle was removed and the wire upsized to accept the sheaths. It was really fairly simple to do (but don't try this at home, I need the work). These sheaths are typically about 1/10th of an inch in diameter, so they are really small, but bigger than a typical IV. The sheath, which has a valve on the end to keep blood from dirtying my shoes, provided an easy roadway to advance catheters through the bloodstream to the heart.

Using x-ray and other imaging, multiple catheters were then inserted in the heart. Multiple catheters were necessary to allow viewing and pacing from different heart locations, mostly for diagnosing the problem before the actual ablation treatment began. So, I inserted a four-pole (quadripolar, there is that rule of longer words again) catheter into the right atrium, the first heart chamber that blood returns to. This allowed me a little window on the atrium, visualized by electrical signals, not actual pictures (though I could see it on x-ray). Similarly, through the other sheaths, catheters were inserted into the right ventricle and the tiny coronary sinus.

The coronary sinus is a little-known secret way to record from the left heart with less trouble. Just as all blood vessels

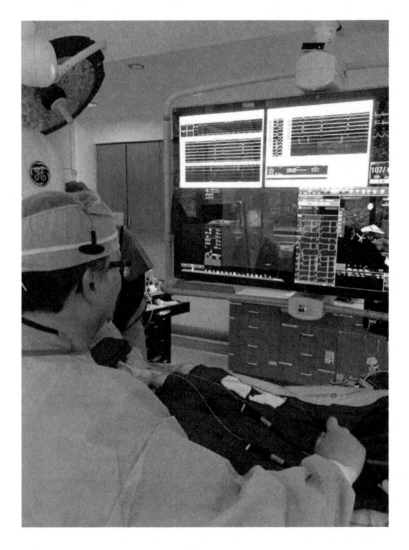

Figure 14.12: A typical EP lab setup for an ablation. The patient's head is to the left. The handsome EP doc is able to simultaneously review images of EKGs, x-rays, a 3D map of the inside of the heart, and others on a large flat-panel monitor.

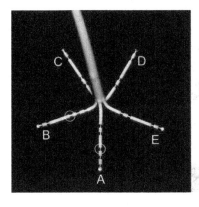
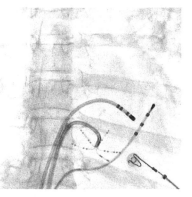

Figure 14.13: A close-up view of a PentaRay catheter, which can collect electrograms from 20 electrodes simultaneously. A fluoroscopic image of an ablation showing a PentaRay, a coronary sinus catheter and the larger tip ablation catheter (arrow). (With permission, Biosense Webster).

everywhere, we have arteries that carry oxygen to our body (hence the pulse in your wrist), and right alongside, we have veins, which gather up the "used" blood from their destination to return it to the heart and lungs. The coronary sinus is the vein draining the heart arteries.

In Lisa's case, I also inserted a small sheath into the right femoral (groin) artery for an additional catheter to the left ventricle. This sheath had a dual benefit because it allowed the anesthesiologist and me to watch the exact blood pressure of each heartbeat, called an arterial pressure line. Finally, I inserted the largest sheath, 9 French, in the right femoral vein.[5] This large sheath is really only about 1/10th of an inch across but big enough that it necessitates care when removing it so you don't spring a leak. Thus, when we were all done, the sheaths were pulled while Lisa was asleep and pressure held for at least 10 minutes or longer until safe.

Through the large sheath, I advanced the ablation catheter into the heart. This is an amazing piece of technology. The ablation catheter, like the others, is a steerable wire with electrodes on it to allow us to "see" the heart's electrical activity wherever it is as well as pace from the exact location the catheter touches. It is steerable because of miniscule wires within it attached to a handle so it can curve wherever I need it to go. The ablation catheter also has a large, 4 millimeter or about 1/4 of an inch, electrode at the end to allow RF ablation energy delivery to the heart. At first this catheter is used for mapping, and after you locate the right spot, zapping.

[5] Like most people, doctors like to belittle the French, so we measure sizes in French, which is about 1/100th of an inch.

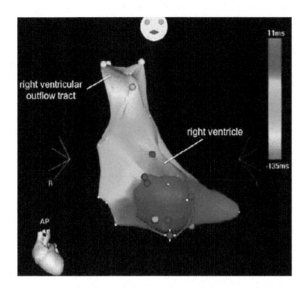

Figure 14.14: 3D elec-
troanatomic maps of heart
chambers for an ablation of
PVCs and VT (With permis-
sion, Biosense Webster).

14.4.1   *Mapping the heart*

Finally, we are ready to map the heart. For arrhythmias, there
are several types of mapping. First of all, you need to do a 3D
electroanatomic map of the heart chamber's interior to know
where it is and so you don't have to use x-ray all the time.

I often give my patients a colorful copy of the map after the
case is over to help explain what was done as well as to ease
the pain of the bill they will receive for work done while they
were sleeping. Mapping can be done in regular sinus rhythm,
or you can also do it while the patient is in an arrhythmia. Lisa
had an easily inducible VT, so I did both location mapping and
also point mapping to define where the trouble started. In her
case, I temporarily replaced the ablation catheter with a mul-
tipole PentaRay® catheter. The PentaRay has five legs, which
reminds me more of an octopus than a PentaRay, whatever that
is.

Regardless, these five legs are very soft, but when mapped
by a fast computer, they allow us to simultaneously collect 20
points and measure their timing. In VT, Lisa's blood pressure
would get really low after a minute or so and my anesthesiologist would very politely warn me to "stop it!" The ability to
map 20 sites at once saved time and risk to Lisa. She stabilized
and I would bring VT on again, mapping until either the anes-

thesiologist cried "uncle" or the map was complete. This is why you want to be asleep. You are better off not knowing. Trust me, I'm a doctor.

With the assistance of the PentaRay catheter, I was able to collect about 500 points in Lisa's right ventricle in less than 5 minutes. In VT, her heart rate was about 165 beats a minute, so one beat lasted about a third of a second. The 3D mapping computer was able to look at signals and time them with this fast heartbeat so we could measure in milliseconds (Pig Latin for miniature seconds). Because these small differences are hard to see, each of the 500 points is colored so you can easily figure out which part of the heart starts the VT earliest.

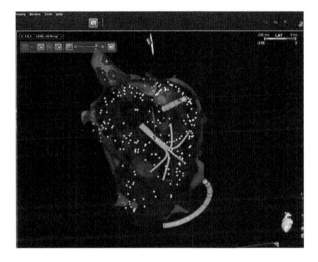

Figure 14.15: With modern mapping technologies, the catheter registers its location on a color map of the heart's interior helping to pinpoint the arrhythmia's origin (With permission, Biosense Webster).

Essentially, that is all there is to mapping, this latter type with colors is called activation mapping. Using the geographic map of the ventricle's anatomy and overlaying the colored map to time the part of just one fast heartbeat, you define the point of earliest activation. Using this technique, the site where Lisa's VT started was accurately identified.

Safely back in regular rhythm, I removed the mapping catheter and placed the ablation catheter back in Lisa's right ventricle, all through the groin sheath. Using the 3D map we created, which can be rotated on the monitor to show any an-gle, I placed the ablation catheter right next to the target area. The newest ablation catheters even have tiny pressure sensors at their tips to give feedback about whether I press too softly or too firmly at the spot selected. I have no idea how they get regular electrodes, ablation electrodes, steering wires, pressure, and temperature sensors into this tiny catheter, which is about 1/10th of an inch across. There must be some really tiny elves that do it and they don't come cheap. Just one of these catheters costs about $2,000.

When all was ready, the ablation energy was delivered.

14.4.2   *Ablation delivery*

Think of ablation as "phasors on stun." As mentioned, after the demonstration of the risks of DC ablation, EP doctors frantically found a less dangerous energy source. Today, the most common energy source remains RF ablation, though we also sometimes use cryoablation. RF is actually a type of energy that heats the tissue without getting the catheter tip warm, though we still call the lesions we create a *burn*.

An RF burn damages only about 1/10th to 1/4th of an inch of heart tissue, about the size of two to three letters on this printed page. The ablation burn is so little you can't even measure any damage to the heart by current tests. However, leaving the skeleton of the heart intact (an actual term we use for the backbone of the heart cells), the electrical activity of these bad boys is destroyed.[6] Typically, you need to leave the RF energy on for 30 to 120 seconds at each spot and you might need to burn from 10 to 50 different spots to cure the arrhythmia (EP doctors with the glasses and years of radiation clouding their eyes are really bad shots).

When you are all done, you get a nice color picture of the heart with these red dots on it showing the ablation locations. More importantly, if done right, you cure the arrhythmia.

As mentioned, Lisa had VT that was potentially life-threatening, confirmed by her low blood pressure when in VT while lying flat in the safety of the EP lab. Imagine how bad this could be if her VT happened while driving on the freeway. Before the ablation, I could easily start her VT and it would stay at 165 bpm until I stopped it by shocking her chest, like the paramedics do. This approach sounds bad but it is routine and just one more reason you want to be sound asleep for your ablation. After the

[6] Now, it isn't as simple as a videogame or we couldn't charge all that money. To be honest, sometimes it is more fun than a videogame when you can watch in 1 second an arrhythmia disappear and really help someone.

ablation, try as I might, I could no longer cause Lisa's heart to race. Remember that surgical expression, "A chance to cut is a chance to cure?" Just substitute *burn* for *cut*.

After we were done, which typically is 2 to 3 hours later, and were comfortable the arrhythmia was fixed, we undid everything. The catheters came out, then the sheaths, which required hand-held pressure until the bleeding stopped. Next, the anesthesia was lightened and the breathing tube was removed. The patient was carefully transferred to a gurney and transferred to the Post Anesthesia Care Unit. We used to call this unit the recovery room but people could understand that so we came up with a more confusing name, see rule number one in medicine.[7] Typically, a patient wakes up gradually and is ready for discharge in 4 to 5 hours.

[7] Rule number one: Medical words must be longer than normal words.

14.5   Robotic ablation

Robots are increasingly common in medicine today. Not the Jetsons' maid type (remember Rosie?) but as tools to assist physician activities. For example, more robotic prostate surgeries are now performed than open surgical procedures.

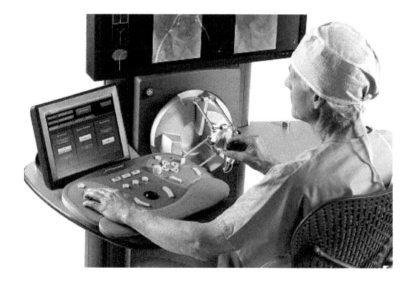

Figure 14.16: Catheter Robotics Amigo Remote Catheter System (With permission, Catheter Robotics).

In EP, we have had several types of robotic assistance available since 2005. Available systems include:

- The Stereotaxis Niobe II magnetic navigation system

- The Hansen Medical Sensei® robotic sheath

- The Catheter Robotics Amigo Remote Catheter System

At Scripps, we have the latter two systems. To be honest, less than 5% of ablation procedures are currently robotic-assisted because the technology is still relatively primitive. As a result, the benefits, whether measured in time savings or radiation reduction, remain unproven. However, we still hear that robots will be common in the future (at least that's what Siri keeps telling me).

14.6   Wrap: What to expect after your ablation

An enormous hospital bill. Seriously, even if you come and are discharged the same day, hospitals can charge more than $100,000 for an ablation, 2 to 3% of that going to the doctor and the doctor's team (see why I must write a book?). Typically, insurance pays about $20,000 or less and the hospital writes off the rest. You will only get charged based on how your insurance works, the average person paying $2,000 or less. Don't forget to negotiate with the hospital if they get paid well by insurance and you still have a large unpaid portion due.

Immediately after your ablation you will awaken in a recovery room; it might be disorienting, but quickly you will be back to normal. The pain is often minimal to nonexistent. After all, you only had a big IV in your groin, not your chest cracked. Sometimes, patients do feel chest pain hours or a few days after from the actual ablation burns in your heart. This is not a heart attack. It is due to inflammation and actually gets better with anti-inflammatories (NSAIDs like Advil) rather than narcotic pain pills.

You will be forced to stay at bedrest for 4 to 6 hours after an ablation to make sure the holes in your groin vessels seal over enough that you won't spring a leak. Minor bleeding is common and can result in a small bruise that clears in the next few weeks. As the blood from the bruise clears, it often forms a multi-colored design as it spreads to the skin. I tell patients that this is like spilling gasoline on the garage floor, a little spreads a long way before it evaporates.

Back to what to expect after your ablation. We covered your bill, chest pain, and groin issues. There isn't much else other than your arrhythmia. No ablation has a 100% success rate, so there is always a concern about a recurrence. Typically this happens in the first few weeks post ablation—most patients have more SVEs and PVCs after an ablation. We used to wait 3 months to officially pronounce every ablation patient cured, but that step is skipped today because it's usually evident. One exception is AF ablations. It's not uncommon to have some actual AF post ablation that is often ignored unless it continues after 3 months.[8]

The real problem post ablation is that you have spent the last several months to years knowing your heart would race at any moment. As a result, you have learned to feel your own skipped beats (SVEs, PVCs) knowing that these can cause your heart to start racing. This conditioning is why the biggest challenge post ablation is to unlearn that feeling. Usually, time will make patients less concerned about normal skipped beats. However, sometimes that biofeedback approach (tell yourself out loud that "this is normal") is necessary. Of course, documentation of your actual rhythm, either with your own monitor, like an AliveCor Kardia™, or one from the doctor's office, can help clarify whether the arrhythmia has reoccurred or is just in your mind.

[8] A man underwent an urgent ablation procedure in a Catholic hospital. In the recovery room, he was visited by a nun. The nun asked him how he expected to pay for his hospital care. She asked, "Do you have insurance?" "I'm sorry, no," he replied in a groggy voice. She insisted, "Don't you have any relative who could help pay?" He stated, "I only have a spinster sister who is also is a nun." The nun, obviously perturbed said, "Nuns are not spinsters! We are married to the Lord." A little more awake, the patient then responded, "OK, then. Send the bill to my brother-in-law."

15
Safety and ablation

There are issues you should learn about before your ablation or, really, any EP procedure, including device surgery.

15.1 Pick an experienced center

If you have read this far, you certainly know that I am a strong advocate of choosing a physician and hospital that has high volume. Complications occur everywhere, but volume makes it easier to prevent as well as easier to rectify. It doesn't matter the procedure, the hospital and doctor should be doing it routinely.

After another medical publication confirmed this link, *U.S. News & World Report* reported the same idea in a 2015 story:[1]

> Like other hospitals in thinly populated areas, Sterling Regional Medical Center does a bit of everything. The 25-bed Colorado hospital has its own heliport, delivers about 200 babies a year and admits more than 1,200 patients for a variety of conditions and procedures. Replacing worn and painful hips and knees is among them. To patients, the surgery might seem perfectly routine.
>
> Joint replacements are anything but routine at hospitals that don't do many of them, a new *U.S. News* analysis shows. Sterling is among thousands of U.S. medical centers whose patients face a greater risk of death and complications because their surgical teams do too few procedures, even common ones, for doctors, nurses and technicians to maintain their skills. And while the death rate for these operations is about 1 in 1,000 nationally, Medicare data in the *U.S. News* analysis show that the relative risk of death for the hospital's elective knee replacement

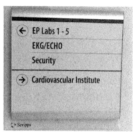

Figure 15.1: Choose a program with high volume, multiple EP doctors and labs (With permission, Scripps Health).

[1] Sternberg, Steve and Dougherty, Geoff. "Risks are high at low-volume hospitals." *U.S. News & World Report*, March 2015.

patients was 24 times the national average and three times the national average for hip replacement patients.

Need I say more?

15.2   Anesthesia

Should you have general anesthesia or conscious sedation?

For ablations in particular, the practice varies from one hospital to another. At Scripps, we use general anesthesia provided by a physician anesthesiologist, though others use competent nurse anesthetists for the same role. General anesthesia means that you are asleep enough that your airway needs protection. The other types include local anesthesia (numbing medication injected at the surgery site, patient remains awake) and an intermediate version, called monitored anesthesia care or moderate sedation (when you get some sleeping medicine intravenously but are still sort of awake). General anesthesia used to always require an endotracheal tube, which crossed the vocal cords and often caused a sore throat and hoarseness post-op.

Today, the most common choice for general anesthesia during shorter (2 to 4 hour) procedures is a laryngeal mask airway (LMA). This brilliant invention, first used in the 1990s, is a soft internal mask that seals the windpipe from any leakage from the food tube or other problems yet allows oxygen to inflate the lungs without the need for an internal airway, the endotracheal tube.

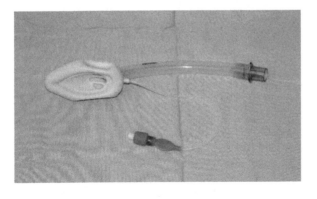

Figure 15.2: A typical laryngeal mask airway (LMA).

An LMA isn't for everyone, particularly if you are overweight, which makes everything we do in medicine just a little bit harder. **Note:** Do not tell your anesthesiologist what type of anesthesia you want. It is fine to discuss your options but that person is the expert. While these MDs might acquiesce to your wishes, I'd recommend allowing them to make the decision about your best care and happiest result.

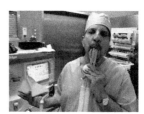

Figure 15.3: An anesthesiologist demonstrating insertion of an LMA on himself (With permission, Syed S. Mahmood, MD).

Anesthesia types vary from hospital to hospital; many other electrophysiology (EP) programs use nurse-monitored, EP-physician-directed IV moderate sedation with potent intravenous medications like Versed (a drug like Valium for amnesia and relaxation), fentanyl (a narcotic like morphine for pain relief and deep sedation), and others. This approach works fine, but my preference is for an anesthesiologist when insurance will pay for it. Not only are the patients happier after general anesthesia, the presence of this competent expert allows me to do my job without distraction. Studies have shown that general anesthesia is actually much safer than moderate sedation used in EP cases.

Unfortunately, general anesthesia has received a bad rap. Most of it is undeserved. First of all, for generations, surgeons too often have blamed anesthesia for post-op issues, thus absolving their involvement (Hey docs, you were the one who did the procedure, man up). It is true that general anesthesia is not without risks, but it is far preferable to the risks without good sedation. Modern anesthesia really is low risk with new, far safer drugs. These new drugs wear off quickly post-op leaving few, if any, side effects so patients routinely go home the same day.

The safety of modern anesthesia was finally gaining traction with the public until two highly publicized celebrity events. Both Joan Rivers and Michael Jackson died from incidents related to anesthesia. Both involved propofol.

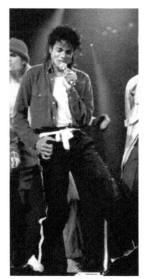

Michael Jackson nicknamed the drug "milk" because apparently he took it every night before bed to help him sleep and it appears as a milky white liquid. As you undoubtedly remember, Michael Jackson died from propofol, administered by an idiot cardiologist (not an anesthesiologist) so this coddled pop icon could sleep at night. In Michael's case, propofol was administered by Dr. Conrad Murray, who was later found guilty of involuntary manslaughter in the case of Jackson's death. For more than 2 months in Michael's home, with limited

Figure 15.4: Michael Jackson performing in 1988 (Photo by Drew H. Cohen/Wikimedia).

medical monitoring equipment, the doctor administered this IV anesthetic agent. On the night of his death, Dr. Murray was distracted and didn't notice that Michael had stopped breathing and aspirated his dinner. A real anesthesiologist would never administer propofol unless you have an empty stomach or it was a real emergency.

Then, there was Joan Rivers. Another idiot non-anesthesiologist (get the trend here?), this time an ear, nose, and throat doctor was evaluating Joan for a hoarse voice. Not even authorized to work at this clinic, Joan brought along this doctor to help the regular doctor because she was self-advertised as the "patron saint of Broadway singers."[2] Without privileges or obtaining consent, the "saint" decided to stick a small scope in Joan's mouth and perform a biopsy (cut a small piece out) on her hoarse vocal cords. Just before this, again without permission, she took a selfie of herself working on Joan to add to her collection. Between the scope in Joan's airway and IV anesthesia administered without proper monitoring, problems developed. Joan didn't get adequate air to her lungs, her heart stopped, and that was it for her too. Pretty sad.

In the hands of a trained anesthesiologist, propofol is a very safe drug. In the cases of both Joan Rivers and Michael Jackson, it wasn't propofol that killed either of them, but medical stupidity. This definitely falls into the advice-your-mother-gave-you category, "Don't do stupid things."

The lessons here:

- Make sure that you are treated just like everyone else, whether you think you are a VIP or not.

- Trust in experience (How many of these have you done?).

- Avoid idiots.

[2] A man approaches his priest with a request. "Father, as you know, my brother Joe just died and I would like you to do the funeral. If possible, can you please mention that he was a saint?" The priest says, "I'll do my best, but I must be truthful in all that I do." At the funeral, the minister begins, "Joe had many challenges in life; he got mixed up with the wrong crowd, went to prison twice, had a drug habit, and offended many. But, compared to his brother, he was a saint."

15.3 Complications

Every medical procedure has some risks. Your job, as well as your doctor's, is to evaluate whether the potential benefit outweighs the risks. No one has a crystal ball, so the best you can do is use statistics to help. Take AF ablation for example: if 100 patients have a pulmonary vein isolation (PVI) ablation and

60% are cured, yet 1 to 6% might have a serious complication, is that risk worth it to you? Part of that decision depends on what the complications could be. One large study of nearly 100,000 atrial fibrillation (AF) ablation patients from 2000 to 2010 found complication rates in order of severity:[3]

- Vascular 1.5%

  - Chest or groin pain

  - Large bruise/hematoma, need for a blood transfusion

  - Arteriovenuos fistula or pseudoaneurysm that might require vascular surgical repair

- Neurological 1%

  - Transient ischemic attack (mini stroke)

  - Stroke with permanent motor impairment

- Cardiac 2.5%

  - Tamponade (fluid around the heart requiring drainage)

  - Atrio-esophageal fistula (hole between the food tube and the heart, you don't want this)

- Death 0.5%

This study found a complication rate of 6.3%, higher with physicians who perform 25 or less a year or in centers doing 50 or less a year (stop me if you have heard this before). Final advice, avoid the doctor who says, "With my luck lately, I'd say your chances are 50/50."

In an attempt to minimize these risks, several recent advances have helped in particular to make AF ablation safer:

- Reduced radiation protocols

- Esophageal temperature monitoring with new multi-electrode catheters

- Early esophageal stent insertion when appropriate

- Echo monitoring for tamponade

[3] Deshmukh, Abhishek et al. "In-hospital complications associated with catheter ablation of atrial fibrillation in the United States between 2000 and 2010." *Circulation*, 128:2104-2112, September 2013.

- Proceeding to full anti-coagulation to minimize stroke risk; don't stop your warfarin or novel oral anticoagulant (NOAC)

Before proceeding, I always tell my patients that no one can predict who will get a complication, so each patient should be willing to look back and remember that they felt bad enough from their arrhythmia to justify the risks. Thus, most that proceed with an ablation are symptomatic, so much so that the arrhythmia is affecting their daily lives.

15.4   *Time-out checklists*

Right after WW II, test pilots were noted to be crashing especially complicated experimental planes at an alarming rate. Surprisingly, investigation uncovered that the accidents were due to foolish mistakes the pilots were making—for example, forgetting to put down the landing gear. And these were our best test pilots. They were so distracted with the complexities of the new planes, they overlooked the obvious.

The Federal Aviation Administration (FAA), and pilots everywhere, then mandated a pre-flight checklist for items that are routine but occasionally overlooked. In 2009, U.S. Airways Flight 1549 made an unpowered landing in the Hudson River after multiple bird strikes caused both engines to fail. Captain Chesley "Sully" Sullenberger attributed his routine checklist in guiding the plane down safely and successfully.

It took until about 10 years ago for us to adopt this safety checklist in medicine. Dr. Atul Gawande, a surgeon from Boston, was the instigator behind this. In 2008, when his research team introduced a "time-out" protocol to eight hospitals, major surgery complications dropped 36% and deaths 47%.

During an ablation procedure or device implant, there are about six to eight medical staff in the room aside from the patient. Before every case the team stops what its doing and first listens to the head nurse and then to the doctor discuss unique aspects about the patient as well as potential concerns. This includes:

- Name with wristband confirmation (I hate it when I operate on the wrong guy)

- Consent signed

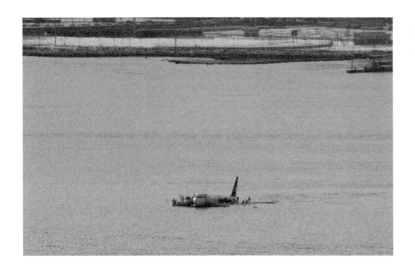

Figure 15.5: U.S. Airways flight 1549 landed in the Hudson River by Captain Sullenberger (Photo by Greg Lam Pak Ng/Flickr).

- Anesthesia provider and type

- Planned procedure

- Special equipment needs

- Allergies

- Site confirmation, right or left (fortunately, we have only one heart)

- Pre-operation preventive antibiotics

- Additional prep needed, such as a Foley catheter or esophageal temperature probe

- Lab results, particularly kidney function if contrast administration is planned

- Additional risks or concerns

- Miscellaneous, such as will a blood transfusion be needed?, what is the fire risk?, and so on

- Post-op anticipated issues (going home, to a hospital room, or to the Critical Care Unit)

- Family notifications (who is in the waiting room, who needs to be updated?)

- Does anyone else on the team have anything to add?

This team aspect is critically important. It takes a village of trained staff all working together for a good outcome. An experienced staff is one of the main reasons why high-volume centers have better results, even when lower-volume doctors perform a procedure.

For the time-out protocol, some centers actually have every team member state their name and role for this procedure. It helps build a team commitment for patient safety. The time-out usually takes no more than 2 to 3 minutes. Initially, some doctors were resistant to the delay necessary to do a proper time-out, complaining, "I'm doing the same exact thing I've done 100 times before." Adding to their cynicism, items like the fire risk are honestly silly for most modern OR situations (you watch now, a fire will break out tomorrow during a case of mine). However, doctors and staff have been won over and we realize that simple points can be overlooked. Safety first.

15.5   The EP team

Who is on a typical EP team?

In the EP lab itself, there are a minimum of two physicians (one EP doctor and one anesthesiologist), although sometimes more. In addition, there will be a couple of cardiovascular technologists or radiology technologists (called techs or "You, over there ...") who might sterilely scrub with me to help with the procedure (don't worry, the docs do all the dangerous stuff, although that might not reassure you by now). There is at least one specialized registered nurse (RN) in the room helping with medication administration and documenting every step of the procedure so the lawyers can find fault later on. It pains me to see how much time nurses now spend documenting on a computer instead of really caring for patients.

In the adjacent room, the control room, are more staff. We use headphones to communicate with the control room because it looks cool and also to minimize the radiation exposure to the staff. When not telling jokes or singing, we discuss over the microphone each aspect of the individual monitors in the control room.[4]

[4] Joe drives home from work on the same route every day, usually after stopping at the pub. Driving on the freeway, Joe's cell phone rings, "Honey, are you on the freeway coming home? I just heard on the news that there is some idiot driving the wrong way down that road." Joe responds, his speech a little slurred, "Thanks, honey, but there ain't just one, there's hundreds of 'em."

In one of our EP labs, I actually counted 16 monitors, and none of them get ESPN. First, there is equipment to run the x-ray. Next to it is the recording equipment, which displays both the recorded and real-time images collected from each electrode pair of every catheter. Next, the complex 3D mapping system is run by an ablation nurse or specialist. In the procedure room (essentially an OR) where I am at the tableside still in a sterile gown, I have a large flat-panel TV to view all the action. It costs about 100 times what the exact same one would at Costco. On it, in sections, each image can be viewed simultaneously, the 3D color map in two views, the stored and live x-ray images, the stored and live EKGs from multiple views for each heartbeat, and the anesthesia monitor showing vital signs.

15.6   Wrap: Patient safety initiatives

The accrediting commission for hospitals, The Joint Commission: Accreditation, Health Care, Certification (also called JCAHO or "JACO"), has made patient safety their major area of focus. By the way, if your hospital is not JCAHO Gold Seal certified, run, don't walk to another one. While TJC imposes a lot of unnecessary regulation on hospitals, it is better than no regulation at all. Mandated measures to improve patient safety have included:

- Avoid abbreviations ("MS" can mean morphine sulfate or mitral stenosis, which is it?).

- Infection control: Publish central line and Foley catheter-related infections.

- Use time-out protocols in surgery.

- Avoid patient falls. (Duh...)

- Encourage patients to discuss their issues (you have a safety role here too).

The elimination of the Latin abbreviation thing took a while for doctors to adopt because that was part of the cool thing about being a doctor, we had a secret language. Plus, it is a lot easier to write "STAT" than "Now." Err...anyways...sometimes the abbreviations are easier.[5]

[5] The famous writing guide, Strunk and White's *Elements of Style* states, "Don't be tempted to buy a $20 word when a fifty center will do." Medical terminology could stand to follow that guide. Of course, Strunk also states rule number one in writing a book is don't personalize the story. Too late.

A few years ago, one of my respected colleagues organized a safety session for catheter and EP lab staff. In it, he had them role-play two different scenarios, complete with different staff members (techs and nurses) acting as a patient, doctor, and others on the team in a typical case. Scenario number one involved good communication between staff and the doctor, "Doc, I see the blood pressure has just fallen. Could that catheter have caused a problem?" This fictional issue was promptly corrected avoiding harm to the patient. Scenario two was identical, except it began with the doctor shouting, "I'm not interested in that ridiculous time-out! Don't bother me; I'm in a hurry!" When this fictional patient's blood pressure dropped to dangerous levels, the staff whispered to each other, afraid to speak up. You can guess how this turned out. This type of team-building exercise really translated into better care. In addition, we learned that some of our staff could easily find another career in Hollywood.

Hospital regulations require a wheelchair for patients being discharged. However, one student nurse had trouble from an elderly gentleman, already dressed holding his suitcase, insisting he could walk on his own. After discussing the rules, the student nurse convinced him to ride. In the elevator, she asked him if his wife was meeting him at the curb. "I don't know," he replied. "She's still upstairs in the bathroom changing out of her hospital gown."

16
Atrial fibrillation

This one arrhythmia could be an entire book topic by itself. Recently, I presented a "Basics of AF" course to some pharmaceutical sales representatives from a big national firm. My class lasted 8 hours with more than 400 PowerPoint slides. Here, I'll hit the highlights and save you from death by PowerPoint.

AF used to be abbreviated as "A Fib" and not because we fibbed. Today, doctors just call if "AF." Of course, AF could be the abbreviation for atrial flutter too (I use "AFl" for that). Just like congestive heart failure—formerly CHF—is now called HF, atrial fibrillation is now most commonly called AF. This does go against the medical maxim to make everything sound lengthy and confusing, but to sound superior we doctors need to always keep the public guessing.

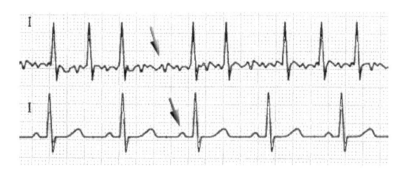

Figure 16.1: EKG comparing AF (top) with a normal rhythm (bottom). The purple arrow on the bottom shows the P wave, which is absent in AF (top). (Image by Jheuser/Wikimedia).

What is AF? AF is an atrial tachyarrhythmia characterized by predominantly uncoordinated atrial activation with consequent deterioration of atrial mechanical function. On the EKG, there is an absence of consistent P waves; instead there are rapid oscillations or fibrillatory waves that vary in size, shape, and timing.

What does this mean in English? This means that your heart rhythm is off for some period of time. It will feel like rapid or irregular beating. Common patient descriptions of AF include "butterflies in my chest," "drums pounding" or if you are from the country, "fish flopping." You might experience heart palpitations, fainting, shortness of breath, or chest pain. Of course, many episodes actually present with no sensation at all, requiring EKG documentation to know you are in AF.

The risk is that these periods of AF can get longer and more dangerous in time.

16.1 Causes and types

Although the most common serious arrhythmia, AF is different depending on the patient. Nevertheless, it is useful to classify basic types to help understand this complex disease. First, let's look at the causes:

- Pre-existing valvular heart disease (for example, a narrowed aortic valve puts pressure on the backstream atria, resulting in enlargement and AF)

- Pre-existing heart failure (weak heart muscle)

- Other recent heart issues, like open heart surgery or pericarditis

- Idiopathic AF (idiopathic is doctor Latin for "we don't really know why.")

This information matters because the treatment might be different depending on the cause. If your valve is diseased, your AF might get better after the valve is repaired. Also, if you have valvular heart disease, anticoagulants don't protect you from stroke as they do in non-valvular AF. Thus, all AF patients are not equal. Regardless, AF is first commonly classified by its duration:

- Paroxysmal or intermittent, comes and goes and is defined as less than 7 days, usually resolves within a few hours to a day.

- Persistent, remains more than 7 days and up to a year in length, or it requires a cardioversion.

- Long-standing persistent is more than a year of continuous AF with hopes for correction.

- Permanent, which is also called chronic (when we give up on attempts to correct it).

First of all, you need to remember the old adage "AF begets AF," which must be somewhere in the Bible because who else uses "begets." This means that the longer you are in AF, the more likely you are going to remain in AF.

If you have been diagnosed with AF, get it treated early and often. For example, paroxysmal AF can be more easily cured with an ablation or controlled with medication, whereas when it is permanent, well, it might be permanent.

16.2   Just how common is AF?

AF is an epidemic. It accounts for one-third of all hospitalizations for arrhythmia. There are an estimated 2.9 million Americans with AF today and due to the population demographics, that number will double in 30 years. You see, AF becomes increasingly more common the older we get. We are living longer today, so more of us will live long enough to get AF.

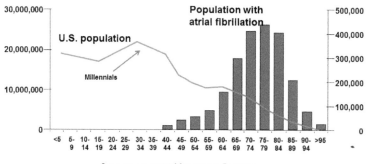

Figure 16.2: The U.S. population gets smaller as we age, with rare increases, such as the baby boomers and the Millennials. As we age, AF becomes more common. (Modified from National Heart, Lung, and Blood Institute).

How your AF affects you makes a big difference in the treatment plans. As is common in about one-half of patients in AF, if you feel a rapid irregular pulse and it irritates you, that is *symptomatic* AF. Others might have the exact same EKG yet not feel it, thus asymptomatic.

Also, the rate of the AF makes a difference. Untreated and in AF, a normal heart goes faster because the atrioventricular (AV) node is bombarded with impulses up to 400 times a minute, so those that get through might make your heart rate (ventricular rate or pulse rate) as fast as 150 bpm. In fact, if you are untreated and your AF has a "normal" rate of say 60 or 70, that means you have AV conduction disease and are headed to a pacemaker someday soon.

16.3 *AF treatments and preventions*

Sir William Harvey first described AF in the 17th century. I guess Bill received his knighthood because he diagnosed AF before the invention of the EKG. Ever since the 1600s, doctors have debated on the best treatment.

In 2004, a landmark study called AFFIRM, involving more than 4,000 patients, looked at the benefits of treatment between two arms:

- **Rate control**, just leaving people in AF but controlling the fast rate with drugs like beta blockers

- **Rhythm control**, more aggressive attempts at anti-arrhythmic treatment and cardioversion in an attempt to maintain normal sinus rhythm

Amazingly, the study found no benefit with aggressive rhythm-control strategies. Cardiologists promptly ignored these findings because it just made sense to try to maintain normal rhythm. Of course, much has changed since then. Because we now have more effective rhythm control medications (for example, amiodarone) and non-medication options (ablation), this might no longer apply. Nevertheless, if you have no symptoms, adequate rate control, and take a blood thinner, it is perfectly reasonable to stay in AF with the rate control option. If it ain't broke, don't fix it.

16.4   Every AF patient needs medication for three reasons

16.4.1   Anticoagulation

The CHADSVasc score discussed in Chapter 11 is an easy way to assess your risk for stroke with AF. Essentially, you need an oral anticoagulant, whether warfarin or the newer novel oral anticoagulants (NOACs), if you have more than one of these seven issues: heart failure, low ejection fraction (EF), hypertension, older than 65, diabetes, prior stroke, and/or you are a woman. Most patients I see have several of these risk factors for stroke. Today, NOACs are often prescribed instead of warfarin.

16.4.2   Rate control

Many of the AF symptoms are actually due to the rapid rate, not the irregularity. Even if you are trying to prevent AF with rhythm control, your AF rate needs to be controlled with an AV node blocker. AV node blockers include:

- Beta blockers (most common today by far)

- Calcium blockers (like diltiazem or verapamil)

- Digoxin (currently in disfavor)

- Others (many anti-arrhythmic drugs like amiodarone and sotalol also have AV node-slowing properties)

16.4.3   Rhythm control

Generally before considering ablation, it is worth trying at least one rhythm control medicine even if it requires a cardioversion (a shock) to get you back in rhythm. The cardioversion will also determine if you feel better when in sinus rhythm. After cardioversion, rhythm control medications maintain sinus rhythm in 40 to 70% of people (at least for a short time).

Anti-arrhythmic drugs include sotalol, amiodarone, flecainide, and others. To avoid serious side effects from the drugs, you should have routine office visits and EKG followups and call promptly if you ever faint.

16.5   What can I do besides drugs?

16.5.1   The importance of weight loss in AF

There isn't a disease (except anorexia) that isn't helped by weight loss, at least until you get down to a normal weight. AF is no exception; in fact your weight is even more important than with most illnesses. So, what is the definition of obese? Morbid obesity means a weight of 270 pounds or higher for an average height person (5'9"). Regular (not the morbid type) obesity begins at 200 pounds. Obesity causes several unique problems in AF:

- Obesity increases your risk of getting AF about 50%.

- In obese sheep (insert joke here), weight loss resulted in dramatic decrease in atrial scarring (fibrosis) associated with AF. Lose weight, less atrial scarring, thus less AF.

- Ablation coupled with weight loss dramatically improves results; 87% cure vs. 48% in the morbidly obese with the same ablation.

- Many EP doctors are reluctant to do an AF ablation on the morbidly obese due to lower success and increased complications.[1]

- In the morbidly obese, bariatric (weight-loss) surgery has been shown to be more successful in treating AF than drugs or ablation.

16.5.2   Other problems that if treated might help your AF

There are many other medical problems associated with an increased risk of AF, what doctors call co-morbidities (which sounds so much more professional than "other problems"). Just like obesity, treatment could prevent or control your AF. These AF co-morbidities include:

- Hypertension (high blood pressure)

- Coronary heart disease (especially a massive prior heart attack)

- Heart failure

[1] Dr. John Day, current Heart Rhythm Society president, used to do three AF ablations a day until he himself got obese and ill. Now he professes weight loss and preloading with water instead. Read his book, *The Longevity Village*, about thin Chinese people who get less AF and live to age 113.

- Enlarged heart chambers for any reason (noted on an echocardiogram)

- Slow heart rates (the slower the heart, the more a single skipped beat can cause AF)

- Valvular heart disease (most commonly aortic stenosis or mitral regurgitation)

- Pericarditis (inflammation of the sack around the heart from a virus or heart surgery)

- Thyroid disease or diabetes (get your blood tested for these)

- Electrolyte abnormalities (such as considerably low potassium)

- Wolff-Parkinson-White (WPW) syndrome

- Lung disease (such as cigarette-related chronic obstructive pulmonary disease or COPD)

- Sleep apnea

Treating these associated problems doesn't always eliminate your AF but it might help.

We discussed alcohol ingestion when talking about cardiac risk factors. Alcohol use is generally *not* a risk factor for increased coronary heart disease or for arrhythmias.[2] Research has shown that alcohol does have effects on the heart's conduction system, but proper clinical studies have failed to associate alcohol intake with an increase in arrhythmias.

In general, if you find something repeatedly causes your arrhythmia whether that is binge drinking, bending over, caffeine, heavy exercise, or that annoying neighbor, then avoid it. Don't forget lesson number four from the first day of med school, "If it hurts when you do that, don't do that."

[2] There is an abnormality called "holiday heart syndrome" where acute intoxication might be associated with an increase in arrhythmias, particularly AF. It is debatable as to whether holiday heart is a real syndrome, but with the fun alliteration, it remains in the medical lexicon.

16.5.3   *Get screened for sleep apnea*

What is the best thing you can do to minimize AF? Yup, lose weight. AF is more common in those who are overweight, especially if you have sleep apnea. Today, there are simple at-home sleep apnea tests that don't require you spending a night in a sleep lab, such as the WatchPAT™.

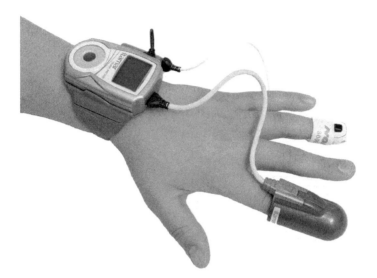

Figure 16.3: The Itamar Medical WatchPAT™ home sleep apnea system (With permission, Itamar).

If you have obstructive sleep apnea and get it treated, usually with a CPAP mask (which makes you look really attractive in bed), the AF might improve or even go away. With CPAP, patients either love it or hate it. Those that have sleep apnea that prevents a normal night's sleep often swear by the system because they awaken re-invigorated for the day.

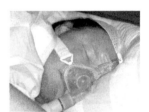

Figure 16.4: Patient using a newer CPAP mask covering only his nose (Photo by Michael Symonds/Wikimedia).

16.5.4   Magnesium

Unlike many other over-the-counter "cures," magnesium is one supplement commonly recommended to treat arrhythmias that actually has some good scientific studies behind it:

- Low blood magnesium (a serum magnesium level of less than 2 mg/dL) increases your risk of AF after open heart surgery by 50%, improved if it is corrected.

- Magnesium is depleted in patients on many diuretics used to treat heart failure, replaced less commonly than potassium.

- Clinical studies have shown that intravenous magnesium has a modest success in converting SVT to sinus rhythm (like verapamil but not nearly as good as adenosine).

Unfortunately, taking extra magnesium when your blood level is normal has never been shown to prevent any serious arrhythmias; but that won't stop vitamin supplement stores from pushing it on you. The MAGICA trial was a randomized double-blind study (that is, real science), which found that large doses of magnesium plus potassium did not decrease AF, SVT, or supraventricular ectopics (SVEs)/premature atrial contractions (PACs). It did decrease patient premature ventricular contractions (PVCs) some, though, without affecting patient symptoms or any other more significant arrhythmia.[3]

My recommendation is to take magnesium only if your serum magnesium is really low (less than 2 mg/dL) and you have symptomatic PVCs. Magnesium comes in lots of forms, a common dose is 400 mg a day of Uro-Mag or Mag-Ox. Otherwise, while it is not harmful, it provides no help. And, for the rest of you, stay out of the vitamin store.

[3] Zehender, Manfred et al. "Antiarrhythmic effects of increasing the daily intake of magnesium and potassium in patients with frequent, ventricular arrhythmias." *Journal of the American College of Cardiology*, 29:1028-34, 1997.

16.5.5   Avoid stimulants

Stimulants cause more SVEs and SVEs make AF more likely to occur. Thus, avoid stimulants, whether that is excess caffeine or cough or cold medicines (and, doctor's orders, stay off the cocaine and crystal meth).

16.5.6   Cardioversion

Cardioversion is the term doctors use for an electric shock to correct a heart rhythm back to normal.

Folklore tells us that the first cardioversion occurred in 1775 when a Danish veterinarian and physician, Christian Peter Abildgaard, who had learned about electricity from Ben Franklin, used a Leyden jar to capture an electrical charge, and applied it to a chicken who promptly fell over dead. Supposedly, Dr. Abildgaard then applied a second charge to the dead bird and he jerked, blinked, and clucked off into the woods.

In a little more scientific approach, Dr. Bernard Lown of Harvard in 1963 used direct current (as opposed to alternating current that comes from the wall socket) shocks on animals after inducing AF with surgery. Lown's defibrillator became a major therapeutic advance. It was not until 20 years ago that the Lown defibrillation waveform was improved into a biphasic shock (a slightly different way to deliver the electricity).

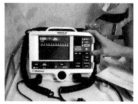

Figure 16.5: After sedation, a cardioversion is performed using a standard defibrillator, converting AF to sinus rhythm (Photo by Alfred Sacchetti, MD).

Today, cardioversions are often coupled with an ultrasound study called a TEE (transesophageal echocardiogram).

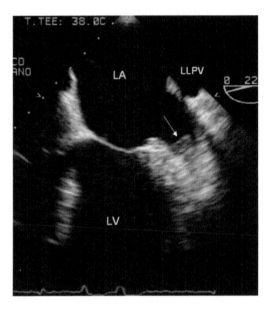

Figure 16.6: Findings from a TEE showing a small clot in the left atrium. It is considered unsafe to perform elective cardioversion when such a clot is discovered because there is an increased risk of dislodgement and brain embolization and stroke.

The TEE helps make sure there is no blood clot in the heart ready to break loose with the shock. Often, taking anticoagulants for 6 weeks or more will dissolve any blood clots rendering a TEE unnecessary.[4]

Cardioversions work in converting AF back to normal sinus rhythm more than 90% of the time. Because the brief electrical shock stimulates the chest wall muscles, cardioversions hurt if you are awake and are typically done with brief conscious or deep sedation.

The real question is how long will the conversion to sinus rhythm last? Anti-arrhythmic medications are often started before your cardioversion to help you maintain sinus rhythm after the shock, but AF recurs more than 50% of the time in the next 6 months. Most importantly, one of the big benefits of conversion is that you will learn if you really feel better or not when out of AF. If you feel better in regular rhythm, it makes sense to proceed with more aggressive treatment options.

[4] The British call a TEE a "TOE" because they spell esophagus with an "O." When will they ever learn proper English?

16.5.7 Ablation for AF

The most common complex ablation procedure today is called a pulmonary vein isolation (PVI) for AF. We have learned that at least for paroxysmal AF, the problem starts in a small area of tissue where veins return blood from the lungs back to the heart. Unfortunately, this is one of the most remote locations in the body to reach. A typical PVI ablation takes 3 to 4 hours or more because catheters have to be inserted across a small hole created in the atrial septum and each pulmonary vein is isolated individually.

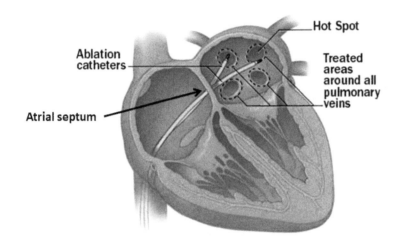

Figure 16.7: Catheters advanced across the intra-atrial septum following a transseptal puncture. The left atrium is mapped and pulmonary veins isolated with ablation energy.

For success, this procedure requires sophisticated mapping equipment with 3D renderings of the inside of the heart, which allows us to register where our ablation lesions have been created.

Like so many things in medicine, AF ablation either works or it doesn't. Personally, I believe that many patients are cured with their first PVI while the others who aren't really don't do that well, even with a redo or focusing on more ablation locations. While nearly every PVI ablation patient leaves the hospital in sinus rhythm, the success rate during the next year is only about 50 to 70%. Maybe someday, the AF ablation outcomes will improve.[5]

Today, ablation for AF is often considered relatively early in AF management, partly due to that "a chance to cut is a chance to cure" mentality and partly due to the fact that results are better with AF that comes and goes (paroxysmal) as opposed to persistent AF. The earlier we can diagnose AF, the better.

[5] AF is such a problem that these lower success rates are acceptable to many, particularly because the best medical therapy has a long-term success rate of 25 to 40%. Sort of damned if you do, damned if you don't.

Presumably, with time, the persistent AF damages (remodels) the atria so that other areas get diseased, such as the rotors described above, and it becomes harder to cure AF with ablation, no matter what you do. Seriously, if you are lucky to be in that group that have an initial success, it is clearly worthwhile because your AF is gone and you don't need medications other than a blood thinner, which can even be stopped eventually for some patients.

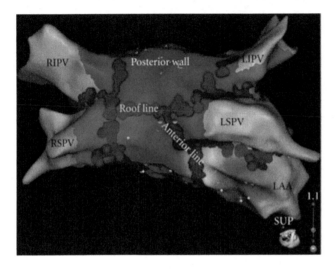

Figure 16.8: An example of the images created during an AF ablation with a 3D rendering of the left atrium, pulmonary veins as well as the lesions (each red dot) where ablation has occurred isolating the veins. (With permission, Biosense Webster).

If the first PVI is done well (confirmed with what is called PVI electrical isolation), yet your AF recurs, carefully consider the possible lower success of repeat ablation balanced with the risks, including the additional radiation exposure. One study, STAR AF 2, found that failures might not benefit from a redo isolation or the roof line. However, another study found that PVI isolation isn't perfect even though proven at the time of ablation number one, so that a redo might improve success.[6] Ablation for AF continues to evolve.

[6] In those whose recurrence is just an atrial flutter arrhythmia (whether from the left or right atrium), repeat ablation might have a better success rate.

16.5.8   AV node ablation

An alternative to a PVI ablation or a redo is called an AV node or AV junction ablation. To be honest, this seems archaic because the point is to intentionally destroy the only electrical connection between the atria and ventricles, rendering the patient pacemaker dependent. However, of all the procedures I do, the AV node ablation patients are the happiest. Why? Because it works. It relieves the symptoms of AF (those butterflies in your chest) plus patients can discontinue most heart medications.

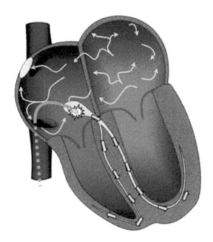

Figure 16.9: An AV node ablation prevents atrial signals from reaching the ventricles but also requires a permanent pacemaker implant (With permission, London Arrhythmia Centre).

The lower heart (ventricles) still beats at a slow rate of 40 or less, so a permanent pacemaker must be surgically implanted immediately after an AV node ablation. As we discussed in the pacemaker chapter, the most common post-AV node ablation pacemaker today is a biventricular one to provide cardiac resynchronization therapy (CRT).

Patients are often concerned about what would happen if their pacemaker stopped. First of all, that is extremely rare because these devices are incredibly reliable. Problems are further minimized by inserting two ventricular leads (right ventricular and left ventricular), providing a "belt and suspenders" type of redundancy in the situation if one lead dislodges.[7]

Often I reserve AV node ablation and pacemaker procedures for those who already have significant bradyarrhythmias (slow heart rates) or for those who have failed prior PVI ablations (a growing group). This is a better option for older people.

Unfortunately, when the AV node is ablated, the atria still silently fibrillate, so patients need to continue their anticoagulation. They just can't feel the AF anymore. I have had some AV node ablation patients come back to the office telling me, "Oh

[7] Even if you get shot in the pacemaker (about as likely as it just stopping without warning), you still have an escape rhythm (typically 30 to 40 bpm), though, you will feel lousy and will require attention to get the pacemaker repaired.

no, I can still tell when I am in AF." Interrogating their pacemaker, I ask them "Well, what is your rhythm now?" Nearly
half the time they are wrong. As I mentioned, most are just
thankful that they can no longer feel the irregularity and rapid
pulse. After all, our goal is to make people feel better.

Even after a successful PVI ablation, it remains controversial
as to whether it is safe to stop anticoagulant medication. Of
course, it does make sense that your risk of stroke must be less
if your AF is truly cured. Some experts argue that the atria are
so damaged from the ablation that the risk of stroke remains
even after a successful procedure. As a result, I encourage both
patient groups to remain on their anticoagulatant medication if
possible. Some who can't take an anticoagulant might look for
alternative options.

16.5.9   *Left atrial appendage occlusion*

Aside from symptoms, the main concern with AF, post ablation or not, is preventing stroke risk. Recently, there has been
a lot of press about a procedure to prevent strokes. This procedure intentionally closes the tiny outpouching in the left
atrium where most heart blood clots originate, the left atrial
appendage (LAA). This is an entirely separate procedure from
an ablation and doesn't do anything about arrhythmias.

The left atrial appendage is a tiny pocket where a clot can
develop when the atria fibrillates. Except for lawyers, more
than 30% of our blood flow goes to our brains. Interestingly,
that number increases when you are concentrating really hard
(like when you are trying to figure out one of my jokes). If
that clot breaks free, it is free sailing to the brain. That is why
strokes are common in AF patients.

Particularly for people who cannot take anticoagulants, such
as those who have bleeding ulcers or other issues, the risk of
stroke must be managed in some other way. A nondrug alternative seems like a good idea if it works. After setbacks
and rejections in 2010 and 2014, Boston Scientific finally received FDA approval for the WATCHMAN™ device in 2015
and promptly went on a PR binge highlighting the device in
the general media. Despite the two prior rejections, the Food
and Drug Administration (FDA) wording was surprisingly le-

nient, eligible patients required standard criteria plus only an "appropriate rationale" to not take warfarin.[8]

Boston Scientific marketed the WATCHMAN aggressively. Unfortunately for them, the other government arm, the payor Center for Medicaid and Medicare Services (CMS), responded like Lee Corso, "Not so fast, my friend." The center approved payment only for those who absolutely cannot take warfarin, not just those who didn't want to take it. It was fascinating that CMS came to a different conclusion than the other government arm, the FDA. Personally, I think CMS got it right for some patients. These left atrial appendage occlusion devices should be limited to those in greatest need only.

[8] As a Boston Scientific representative put it, "You don't really want to take rat poison the rest of your life, do you?"

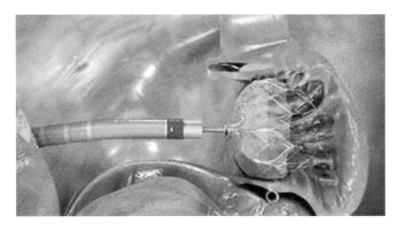

Figure 16.10: Rendering of deployment of a WATCHMAN™ left atrial occlusion device in the LAA (With permission, Boston Scientific).

An alternative to the WATCHMAN, another left atrial appendage occlusion device, the Lariat™, has been available for several years, developed by SentreHEART. It is a snare or noose (like a cowboy's lariat, get it?) that is circled around the left atrial appendage from the outside of the heart. Cleverly, the inventors got the Lariat™ approved only for "soft-tissue approximation" anywhere in the body, like tying off a bleeder in laparoscopic surgery.

When it was approved, physicians adapted it for use in the left atrial appendage with some success, but little scientific testing of safety. Even one of the original investigators stated, "The Lariat™ device is an absolutely ingenious piece of engineering for closing the left atrial appendage; however, ingenuity does not guarantee safety and efficacy."

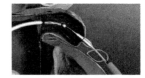

Figure 16.11: A Lariat™ uses magnets and an internal and external approach to lasso the left atrial appendage (With permission, SentreHEART).

Despite never undergoing traditional FDA evaluation, the Lariat™ has been used in more than 4,000 patients, compared to about 1,500 WATCHMANs. When it finally surfaced that Lariat™ LAA closure was associated with an emergent open heart surgery rate of about 2% and mortality of about 0.5%, the FDA stepped in with a warning, but it has not banned this use yet. The concern started with a well titled article by medical writer Larry Husten in *Forbes*, "The Lariat™ Needs Lassoing." I agree with this concern.

16.6   Wrap

So, now you know to call atrial fibrillation AF. What else can you remember?[9] Here's the *Reader's Digest* condensed version:

- AF presents differently in every patient.

  - Some with horrible symptoms, some without any.
  - Some come and go, others last for years.
  - It gets worse as we age, like everything.

- A few things you can do short of ablation.

  - Keep your weight down.
  - Get checked for sleep apnea.
  - Schedule some tests to find out why you have it (echocardiogram and blood work).
  - Lay off the caffeine (and any other stimulants like cough medicine).
  - Keep your weight down (or did I say that?).

- Your stroke risk can be predicted (using the CHADSVasc score).

  - There are newer anticoagulants other than rat poison.
  - There are procedures if blood thinners don't work for you.

- Treatment options depend on your risks and how you feel.

  - Medications
  - Cardioversion (shock treatment)
  - Ablations of several types

[9] In a college town deep in the South, three college students majoring in logic go into a bar. The bartender asks, "Y'all want a beer?" The first one answers, "I don't know." The second one answers, "I don't know." The third one responds, "Yes."

17
Heart failure

Why is there a chapter on heart failure (HF) in a book on arrhythmias?

HF is not only a huge medical problem, it is the most common cardiac condition associated with arrhythmias.[1] Sometimes HF causes arrhythmias, other times arrhythmias cause HF.

In the medical world, heart failure is the term doctors use for the grab bag situation when the heart does not pump effectively. If your heart doesn't pump enough blood, oxygen, and nutrients to your body, you get tired, short of breath, weak, and just plain feel lousy. It comes in two basic varieties:

- *Systolic heart failure*, where the heart is enlarged and each beat ejects less blood

- *Diastolic heart failure*, where the heart is too stiff and can't fill adequately

Depending on how you define it, systolic heart failure is four times more common than diastolic heart failure.[2] It is primarily a problem of thickening of the heart muscle, most commonly from untreated hypertension. While it puts extra stress on the atria and is associated with AF and other arrhythmias, it is generally less of a problem to control.

Commonly, regular or systolic heart failure is further divided into ischemic (from prior heart attack due to coronary artery disease/CAD) or nonischemic (all other causes of heart enlargement and HF). In the United States, ischemic cardiomyopathies comprise about 70% of the causes of HF, though that is 50% in

[1] I found one definition that "heart failure is a medical condition when the heart pump fails." If you think this sounds circular like, "engine failure is a condition where your engine fails," I don't blame you.

[2] Remember, systole is *pumping*, diastole is *filling*.

Europe and about 30% in South America (due to more infections, less CAD, and so on). As I briefly discussed Chapter 7, the causes of systolic heart failure are numerous:

- CAD (prior heart attacks, called ischemic cardiomyopathy)

- Hypertension (causes thickened heart walls and systolic or diastolic HF)

- Valvular heart disease (most commonly, aortic stenosis or mitral regurgitation)

- Viral infection, often from years prior slowly destroying heart muscle (common one)

- Congenital heart disease (born with a defect that leads to HF)

- Infection of a valve, called endocarditis

- Diabetes (usually from heart attacks but also can cause small vessel disease and damage)

- Alcoholic cardiomyopathy

- Drug-induced

  - Chemotherapy drugs, several but not all classes
  - Cocaine and amphetamines (like speed and other uppers)
  - Some anti-arrhythmics (though the worst are off the market now)
  - Nonsteroidal anti-inflammatory drugs (NSAIDs)—even Advil can cause salt and fluid retention)
  - Rare: immune modulators, anti-psychotics, diet drugs

- Tachycardia cardiomyopathy (from consistent fast rates or very frequent premature ventricular contraction/PVCs)

- Pacing induced (from right ventricular pacing only in those pacer dependent)

- Rare postpartum complications due to pregnancy

- Takotsubo cardiomyopathy (broken heart syndrome)

- Other rare conditions from spider bites to HIV to Chagas disease

17.1   Broken heart syndrome

I'll bet you thought that "broken heart" was just a term for melancholy after a breakup.

Not until a decade ago did physicians realize that certain stressful situations are associated with the development of a specific type of heart failure, first called "apical ballooning syndrome." Unfortunately, the medical term that caught on is takotsubo cardiomyopathy, as the ballooning apparently looks like a Japanese octopus trap.

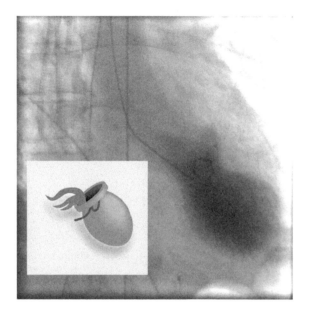

Figure 17.1: Angiogram in a patient with takotsubo cardiomyopathy and apical ballooning compared with a Takotsubo ("Japanese octopus trap") (Photo by Tara C. Gangadhar, Elisabeth Von der Lohe, Stephen G. Sawada, and Paul R. Helft).

About 85% of cases are associated with a very stressful event either emotional (grief, relationship issues, and so on) or physical (asthma attack, surgery, and so on). This is followed by the sudden onset of heart failure symptoms (shortness of breath, fatigue, chest pain) and with EKG findings that often mimic a heart attack. In fact, many patients come in with chest pain and get urgent coronary angiograms to only find that the arteries are normal, but the left ventricle, our heart's main pumping chamber, is bulging at the apex and has a markedly diminished ejection fraction (EF). For some reason, this is increasing in frequency (or at least recognition), now comprising about 2% of so-called STEMI urgent angiograms for heart attack treatment.[3]

[3] STEMI is shorthand for ST-segment elevation myocardial infarction. These are full-blown heart attacks caused by blockage of a coronary artery. ST-segment elevation refers to a the particular pattern that appears on an EKG.

For obvious reasons, takotsubo cardiomyopathy is commonly called broken heart syndrome because that is a lot easier to remember. It is more frequent in post-menopausal women than men (about 70/30). Patients often heal within days to weeks but some develop permanent heart failure, arrhythmias, and go on to need ICDs or even a heart transplant.

So as mom taught us, "Remember to be kind to each other."

17.2   Congestive heart failure

The old term for systolic congestive heart failure is CHF. Today, because doctors are always trying to make things less complicated for patients, we just call it heart failure or HF. When the left ventricular pump fails to empty of blood, it backs up, raising pressures in the previous chambers. First, the left atrium, then the lungs, and then the right ventricle and right atrium. This elevated lung pressure, called pulmonary hypertension is why HF patients are short of breath. The enlargement of the chambers increases the incidence of numerous rhythm problems, particularly AF, PVCs, and VT/VF, the cause of sudden death.

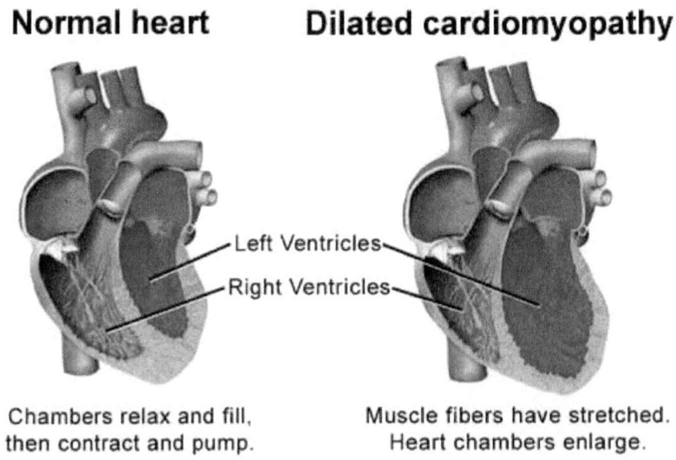

Normal heart   **Dilated cardiomyopathy**

Left Ventricles
Right Ventricles

Chambers relax and fill,
then contract and pump.

Muscle fibers have stretched.
Heart chambers enlarge.

Figure 17.2: Illustration of a how the heart is affected by heart failure. The left ventricle is first to dilate but, with time, the other chambers backstream also dilate from elevated filling pressures, causing arrhythmias (With permission, Bruce Blausen, Blausen.com).

HF often occurs at a baseline with periodic exacerbation, generally after you overeat fast food that is high in sodium, retain water, and then your heart can't keep up. These acute episodes are also associated with an even greater chance of dying from sudden death, or if you are protected by an ICD, of getting a shock.

17.3   HF is worse than cancer

HF afflicts more than 5 million Americans, way more than hemorrhoids and the heartbreak of psoriasis combined (and all cancers too). This includes more than 1% in our 50s but by the time you reach 80, 10% have HF. The death rate in the United States is about 50,000 a year just from HF alone. It presents a tremendous cost burden to our health care system, more than 5% of our entire health care costs or more than $38 billion a year.

Despite all the advances in medicine designed to shorten hospital stays, the average length of an HF stay remains 7.1 days, longer than the average stay for open heart surgery. Forty years ago, when they let you stay in the hospital until you were better (what a concept), the average length of stay was 11.7 days, so we haven't improved that much.

Why is a diagnosis of HF worse than cancer?

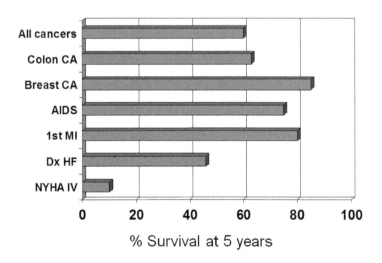

Figure 17.3: Estimated 5-year survival at time of diagnosis with common medical illnesses (Data from CDC).

The figure shown illustrates the 5-year survival rate with

most common cancers as well as other illnesses, like AIDS and heart attack. Advances in cancer treatments have dramatically improved survival rates. However, from the day that you are first told you have heart failure, your chance of being alive in 5 years is 50/50. If you need hospitalization for HF requiring IV medicines, called NYHA Class IV heart failure, that death rate becomes 90% at 5 years and 50% in just 1 year. Isn't that just a ray of sunshine?

Fortunately, there are huge advances in the treatment of HF today, which should impact those depressing statistics. Better treatments for HF mean less arrhythmias, a dual benefit.

17.4 HF treatments

I show patients a slide of a doctor with a bottle of pills larger than he is because there are presently so many medications necessary and helpful for a HF patient. The caption on the slide reads, "I hope you don't have trouble taking pills." Medication classes include:

- Diuretics: Water pills to clear the body and lungs of excess backed up fluid[4]

- Angiotension converting enzyme (ACE) inhibitors/Angiotension receptor blockers (ARBs): Lower blood pressure and encourage the kidneys to function better

- Beta blockers: Slow the heart rate and help it relax

- Spironolactone: A different kind of diuretic that helps the heart function

- Statins: Even those without markedly elevated cholesterol seem to do better with a statin

- Digoxin: As with atrial fibrillation (AF), being used less for HF because risks might outweigh benefits

[4] Common diuretics include Lasix and Bumex. Unlike every other medicine's name, Lasix actually was named for a good reason. It is called that because it "lasts six hours" so remember to take it early, at least 6 hours before bedtime.

Systolic HF is associated with a weak heart muscle as measured by the EF, that percentage of blood ejected with each heartbeat, normal being 55 to 70%.

The best predictor of your risk of death from a ventricular arrhythmia is based on your EF:

- Lower than 50%, see a cardiologist.

- Lower than 40%, ask to see an EP specialist; you should also be taking heart failure medications.

- Lower than 30%, an implantable cardioverter defibrillator (ICD) evaluation is urgently needed.

- Lower than 25%, see a heart failure specialist and an artificial heart (left ventricular assist device or LVAD) could be indicated.

- Lower than 10%, don't buy any green bananas.

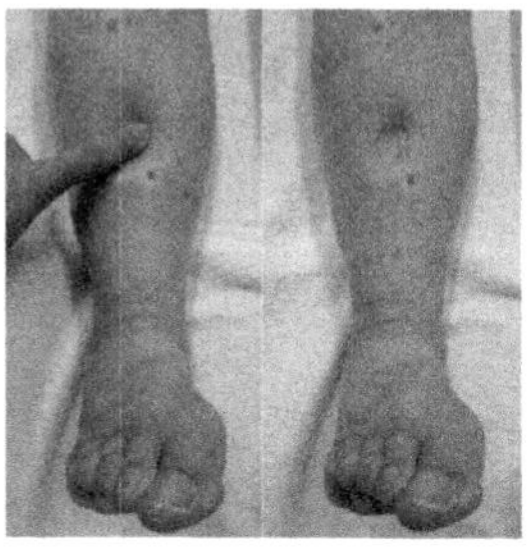

If you do nothing else, taking HF medications alone will improve survival. At the very least, get one of those cheap pill organizers and set an alarm to remind you it is pill time again. However, when medicines alone don't work, there are several amazing recent advances.

Figure 17.4: Pitting edema in a patient with heart failure (With permission, James Heilman, MD).

17.4.1   Cardiac Resynchronization Therapy (CRT)

As discussed in Chapters 12 and 13, the simple (well, not always that simple) addition of a left ventricular lead to resynchronize your heart can improve your survival 25 to 36%.

Although the HF experts don't like to use it, most other physicians still use the NYHA Classification for severity of heart failure:

- NYHA Class I, no symptoms, even with activity (just a low EF)

- NYHA Class II, slight limitation of physical activity, OK at rest

- NYHA Class III, marked limitation of activity, can't keep up with peers

- NYHA Class IV, can't do squat, symptoms occur at rest

These simple criteria have been used to classify patients into various risk profiles. For example, the early ICD studies found the greatest benefit in NYHA III patients, those with bad but not horrible symptoms. Class IV might benefit from an ICD and CRT but often need more help (like a new heart) because

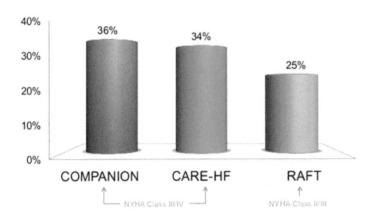

Figure 17.5: CRT can improve your survival rate by up to 36% (Chart adapted from COMPANION, CARE-HF, RAFT studies with permission of authors).

their prognosis remains poor. Fortunately, as the infomercial guy said, "But wait! There's more!"

Since it was first developed, we have since extended this electrical help of biventricular pacing to healthier patients in the NYHA I and II camps. In the MADIT-CRT study, we studied those with mild heart failure—NYHA I or II symptoms. Amazingly, we found that those who got a CRT defibrillator instead of a regular ICD had a 41% reduction in HF hospitalization or death. Thus, although both groups were protected from sudden death with a shock box, the CRT patients with an extra left ventricular lead didn't progress on to severe heart failure as often.

In this group, with zero-to-mild symptoms of heart failure, a low EF (30% in this study) and a wide QRS (greater than or equal to 130), patients dramatically improved with the addition of the left ventricular lead. It is difficult to estimate how many lives this groundbreaking technology has saved.

17.4.2   *Left Ventricular Assist Device (LVAD)*

For those that have Class IV heart failure, sometimes the heart you have just can't be fixed with medication and CRT. In the early days, these pumps tried to duplicate a real heart. Pioneers, such as the first patient ever, Barney Clark, died of stroke complications. In recent years a type of improved artificial heart has made great strides. The LVAD is a small continuously run-

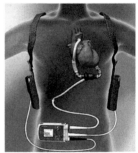

Figure 17.6: An LVAD consists of the pump, implanted in the chest to pump blood from the left ventricle to the aorta, the controller, and battery packs, which reside outside the body (With permission, Thoratec).

ning pump that is implanted in the chest.

The LVAD draws blood from the sick left ventricle and pumps it into the aorta, like a normal heart. There are two FDA-approved LVADs (manufactured by Thoratec and Heart-Ware) that have saved many lives.

Figure 17.6 illustrates that today's pump is a much smaller device. Instead of providing pulsatile flow (up and down), it runs at up to 13,000 rpm thanks to secure bearings made of ruby.[5] These work so well that patients receive them as "destination therapy" meaning they never go on to get a heart transplant. Others, like Dick Cheney, get an LVAD as bridge therapy, just to keep them alive until a transplant is available.

[5] LVADs cost as if they were made of diamonds though, $200,000.

The biggest issue with LVADs is that the batteries are too large to implant, so patients actually have a tube coming through their skin to a battery pack worn as a fanny pack. Infections at that tube site as well as the daily need to change the batteries are major limitations. Likely, technological advances will resolve that concern as happened with pacemakers.

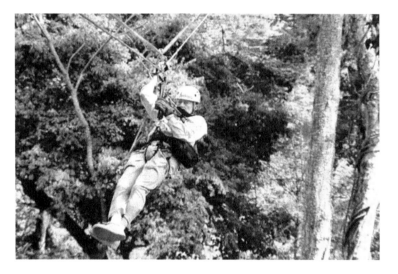

Figure 17.7: A very adventurous LVAD patient enjoying life on a zip line. The battery pack can be seen as his fanny pack (With patient permission, doctor permission for zip lining was not granted).

17.4.3 Transplants

Heart transplants have been around since 1967, first performed in South Africa. Early pioneers included Dr. Michael DeBakey at Baylor in Houston and Dr. Norman Shumway at Stanford University.[6]

[6] Dr. Shumway gave me some of the best advice I ever received, "Never have your picture taken with a drink in your hand. If you don't look perfect, people will assume you were drunk."

Annually, less than 4,000 heart transplants are done world-wide today, about half in the United States. Unfortunately, 2,000 a year is not enough to satisfy the need, with more people dying waiting on the transplant list than actually getting one. One unexpected reason heart transplants remain uncommon is the motorcycle helmet law. After forcing motorcyclists to wear a helmet to protect themselves, there are fewer healthy heart donors available and LVADs are increasingly common. Previous trials evaluated transplanting baboon hearts into humans; the heart worked fine but the patients had incredible cravings for bananas, so that approach was abandoned. You can see why we need research into improved artificial hearts, or perhaps genetic cloning, to develop new ones.

17.5   Wrap

For those of you thinking about zip lining instead of heart failure, here are the highlights:[7]

- HF is the term used for poor heart pumping, causing fatigue and shortness of breath.

- Sometimes HF causes arrhythmias, other times arrhythmias cause HF.

- There are numerous heart failure causes but they are lumped into two groups: those from a prior heart attack and the others.

- HF is more common than cancer (about 5 million Americans affected) with a worse prognosis.

- Treatments include:

   - Medications of several classes. See a specialist.
   - CRT, a left ventricular lead added to a pacemaker or defibrillator that can improve your survival by more than 30%.
   - An artificial heart pump called an LVAD.
   - Heart transplants.

[7] One day, Mr. Jones was playing golf and died of a heart attack. Nobody wanted to tell Mrs. Jones. When Mrs. Jones got worried one of Mr. Jones's friends told her that he lost $5,000 playing poker. Mrs. Jones said he probably dropped dead. "Funny you should mention that," said his friend.

18

Future advances—some available today

Consider these three scenarios from 1995, not much more than 20 years ago:

1. A person alone in his car and talking out loud was considered to be mentally ill and shunned.

2. A person ordering a grande decaf mocha cappuccino was presumed to be speaking Italian.

3. A person standing in a hallway looking down would get a sympathetic look and offer of help.

Of course, today these activities elicit a different response because we take cell phones, Starbucks, and texting for granted. What will life be like in 2035, less than 20 years from now? As the immortal Yogi Berra said, "Predictions are difficult, especially about the future." Think back to 1969 when man first walked on the moon. I am sure prognosticators were convinced that by 2016, we would have huge cities up there. Since 1972, no human has walked or even orbited the moon. Incorrect prediction number one.

In Stanley Kubrick's movie *2001: A Space Odyssey*, the creators predicted in 1968 that computers would be powerful but so massive that HAL (who got his name as one letter back from I-B-M) took up half the space ship. Thanks to the silicon chip, more computer power exists in your mobile phone today. Incorrect prediction number two.

In 1899, the Commissioner of the U.S. Patent and Trademark Office famously said, "Everything that can be invented has been invented." Incorrect prediction number three.

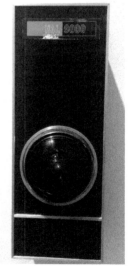

Figure 18.1: The HAL 9000 computer eye from the 1968 film, *2001: A Space Odyssey* (Photo by Carlos Pacheco/Flickr).

Now I feel a little more comfortable making my own medical predictions for the future.

18.1 My personal predictions

1. Pacemakers and defibrillators will no longer have leads.

2. Ablations won't require catheters or x-rays.

3. Gene therapy still won't live up to its hype.

4. Sensors will be everywhere.

5. The *Star Trek* tricorder will be commonplace, able to assess your body's health.

6. You will still be on hold awaiting insurance authorization.

18.1.1 Leadless pacing and defibrillation

In Chapter 12, we discussed the revolutionary leadless pacemakers, the St. Jude Nanostim™ and Medtronic Micra™. They likely will achieve FDA approval soon and, in the interim, remain readily available at research centers like Scripps.

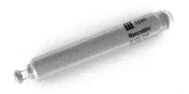

Figure 18.2: The leadless Nanostim™ pacemaker is about the same size as it is on this page (With permission, St. Jude Medical).

Amazingly, once again, just as I was writing this, I stopped for a procedure on just what I am writing about, this time a Nanostim™ implant. I love doing them because these miniature pacemakers are so slick. Start to finish, the procedure took 30 minutes and the patient has no scar, just a bandage on the groin over the venous entry site. This patient had permanent atrial fibrillation (AF), dizziness, and more than 20 documented pauses of up to 4.4 seconds; he will use pacing rarely but needs it to avoid fainting. Leadless pacing is clearly the future of pacemakers, available in limited release now.

The next generation of leadless pacing will involve a dual-chamber system, already in prototype, that includes a second pacemaker for the atrium. Amazingly, the second atrial pacemaker should be even smaller, half the size of the current leadless device. The two leadless pacemaker parts will be able to communicate with each other and a programmer to allow atrial and ventricular pacing. 90% of pacemakers use this feature today. This advance is required before leadless pacing can be available for the masses.[1] A third leadless pacemaker, to be placed through the coronary sinus veins, will be developed to allow cardiac resynchronization therapy (CRT). In fact, a variation on the miniaturization concept has already been developed by Minnesota EBR Systems, which uses an electrode the size of a grain of rice embedded in the left heart and paced by sound waves.

[1] I believe this will happen by 2017 or within a year or 2 thereafter.

Defibrillators require larger batteries and capacitors, so their miniaturization will take longer. As discussed in the Chapter 13, we do presently have a nonvascular implanted cardioverter defibrillator, the S-ICD™, but it is cumbersome and cannot pace except for a few seconds after a shock.

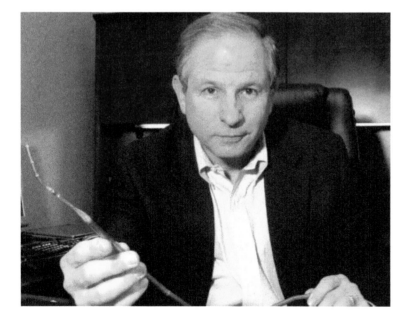

Figure 18.3: Entrepreneur Bill Starling demonstrating the InnerPulse™ implantable ICD and pacemaker (With permission, W. Starling, F. McCoy, Synecor).

An interesting alternative involves an entirely intravascular

ICD, the InnerPulse™ by Synecor. It has no generator, just a large lead with defibrillation coils as well as the brains for the device incorporated in the lead itself. Because this leaves nothing external, presumably there would be a lower risk of infection. Unfortunately, the project currently remains dormant due to regulatory, financial, and technological hurdles. Never fear, leadless defibrillators will be here in the future.

A traditional pacemaker has been called an artificial AV node because it bypasses a diseased conduction area with leads and a generator. What if this could be done with a biological AV node? Studies are ongoing with stem cell infusions and other tissue engineering to restore the heart's electrical function lost to disease. Maybe even leadless artificial pacemakers will be eliminated by this more "natural" approach.

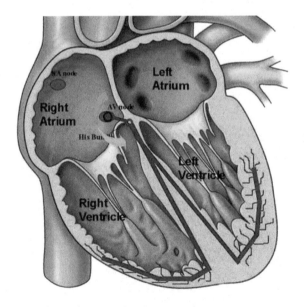

Figure 18.4: Shown in green, a "biological" pacemaker could bypass the AV node and potentially replace the traditional pacemaker.

18.1.2   Ablations without catheters or x-rays

Radiation exposure from frequent computerized tomography (CT) scans, interventional fluoroscopy, and prolonged EP procedures, remains a risk for both patients and medical staff. Magnetic resonance imaging (MRI) technology offers an alternative way to visualize the structures. The very strong magnetic fields associated with MRI have no known risks associated with temporary exposure. However, all the catheters, devices, and current EP lab equipment have ferrous-containing metals in them that make MRI impractical today. Nevertheless, several centers are working on adapting current EP tools for use in an MRI environment. Presently, we already have MRI-safe implanted pacemakers and defibrillators, but we don't yet use MRI imaging for placement.

Our current 3D mapping technology used in nearly all ablations creates images of the heart without the need for x-ray. It is currently possible to do an entire EP and ablation study without radiation using these tools and ultrasound guidance. Some versions (Biosense Webster's UniVu and St. Jude Medical's MediGuide) also store brief x-ray images and superimpose it on the 3D map to help with orientation, and reassurance for us physicians addicted to x-ray images. This can reduce the x-ray exposure by 99%, down from the typical ablation equivalent of more than 1,000 to 2,000 chest x-rays to radiation equal to less than 10.

Even more futuristic would be the ability to do the work without any catheters in the heart. Presently, Scripps is fortunate to have a CyberKnife® robotic radiosurgery system that has replaced some brain surgeries by non-invasively focusing radiation through the skull pinpointed on tumors at various sites in the brain. You can actually have your brain cancer cured in one day without cracking your skull.

A former Scripps heart surgeon, Pat McGuire, has a Bay Area startup, CyberHeart, working on a related concept to use the same CyberKnife® process to focus the lesion on a mapped location in the heart. Theoretically, this could replace catheters altogether.

At last year's Stanford Biodesign symposium, a concept of "Virtual EP" was presented. It uses radiation (Computerized tomography (CT) and fluoroscopy) and MRI images organized by complex computer algorithms to mathematically or "virtually" predict your risk of ventricular tachycardia (VT) or ventricular fibrillation (VF) and sudden death. How amazing would that be? A non-invasive study that could tell you your risk of sudden death and your need for an ICD. If this test is reliable, we could potentially avoid placing defibrillators in patients who

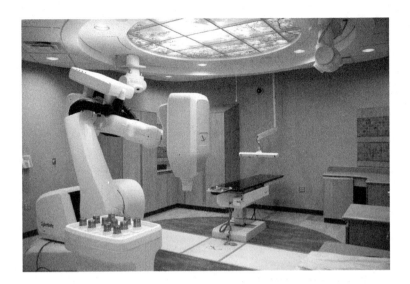

Figure 18.5: A CyberKnife®
focuses radiation to destroy
cancer in the brain, often
in one treatment, with-
out the need for surgery
(Photo courtesy Scripps
CyberKnife Center).

will never use them.

Now, if we can perform EP studies virtually and ablations
by robot, perhaps I might be able to practice from a beach in
Hawaii; that is a future I could get used to!

18.1.3   Genetic advances: Cell and gene therapy

You can't discuss the future of medicine without mentioning
the hope of repairing what directly causes diseases with genetic
advances, called gene and cell therapy. So, what are they?

Cell therapy is an attempt to modify disease by using naturally administered cells, microscopic or barely visible to the
naked eye.

Cell therapy is here now; after all, a simple blood transfusion is cell therapy. A bone marrow transplant is a common
treatment today where damaged or destroyed marrow (with
chemotherapy or radiation first destroying cancer of the blood,
like leukemia and lymphoma) is replaced with healthy bone
marrow stem cells matched to the recipient by blood type. The
new cells are administered by IV and go to the marrow and
reproduce, regenerating the recipient's blood production capability. Even solid organ transplantation, like a heart transplant,
is a form of successful cell therapy.

The future of cell therapy often hinges on stem cell infusions, of which there is much controversy. Embryonic stem cells come from miscarriages or discarded human embryos, illegal in the United States, but they are not necessary for stem cell therapy. Stem cells can be harvested from sources other than embryos, such as umbilical cord blood, or adult stem cells can be grown and reprogrammed to function in many different locations in the body.

To date, no human has ever been cured of any disease using embryonic stem cells. Research is ongoing, especially promising for spinal cord injury and skin grafts for burns. However, there is a dark side. Bogus treatments using stem cells are touted for everything from baldness to erectile dysfunction to arthritis. Because stem cell therapy is not yet approved for any use in the United States, these treatments require a visit to a clinic in other countries. In some stem cell clinics, the treatment of-fered is unproven and of questionable value. Regardless, this hasn't stopped famous celebrities and athletes from seeking the treatment. Buyer beware!

Don't get me wrong, there is legitimate research being done in the United States on non-embryonic stem cells. One promis-ing concept is to replace the scarred heart cells associated with a prior heart attack or heart failure. So far, the results have been marginal at best but research continues. One fun twist was pro-posed to me by a local San Diego company, Cytori Therapeu-tics. They suggested performing liposuction (paid by insurance) to harvest fat from the abdomen, separate out your own stem cells, and then reinfuse them back directly into your heart (or wherever needed). Instead of growing stem cells in a lab, your own harvested cells would be a perfect blood-type match. This could solve two common health problems simultaneously—heart disease and obesity. Wouldn't that be wonderful?[2]

Gene therapy modifies an individual's DNA in hopes of cor-recting an abnormality. Unlike cells, genes are so minute they can't be seen under a microscope.

With recent advances in genome sequencing, some gene abnormalities known to cause diseases are tagged to a specific location on the DNA in one of your 46 chromosomes (23 pairs), located inside the nucleus of your cells. In the near future, it might be possible to correct some of these DNA defects. This could include modifying genes in the sperm or egg stage

[2] By the way, do you know what the most common comment at the liposuction clinic is? "I'm here to get my birthday suit taken in."

or even in utero. Of course, besides the science, this brings up all sorts of ethical issues. While no gene therapy is FDA approved yet, clinical trials are ongoing at many academic centers. I previously mentioned the issues around the home gene sequencing company 23andMe. Unfortunately, much of genetic therapy has been a victim of "over promise and under deliver." Hopefully, this won't always be the case.

18.1.4 Sensors everywhere

NASA conducts an annual design contest for products of the future. Get ready; sensors will be everywhere. Previous winners have included BiancaMed's SleepMinder (now owned by ResMed), a non-contact device that monitors sleep and breathing at home or in the hospital. The BiancaBaby version is an attempt to prevent sudden crib death, which sometimes might be of an arrhythmic origin (long QT syndrome (LQTS) and others).

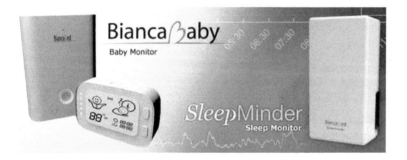

Figure 18.6: Contactless sleep and breathing monitor (With permission, ResMed).

Another NASA winner involved a microwave radar system that can determine some vital signs (respiratory and pulse rate) through a wall. The military is obviously interested in this technology. However, consider the applications for senior care. As our population ages, such systems might allow us to stay in our homes, as a supplement to items that can record heart rhythms and activity level non-invasively and in real time. When granny becomes less mobile, the kids will be notified to check up on her.

Even OnStar®, the GM automobile monitoring company, is getting into health management. They have proposed a system to keep track of humans and notify family or authorities when

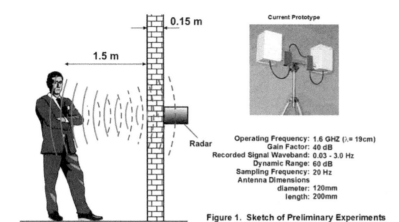

Figure 18.7: BioRASCAN microwave radar for non-invasive vital sign detection.

problems are detected (such as when keys are accidentally locked in your stomach). Proposed features include:

- Non-implanted diagnostics (vital sign and activity monitors)

- Wireless weight and blood pressure management

- Wireless toilet sensors (Really...for urine output and sugar content)

- Wireless motion detectors, GPS, and activity trending

- Automatic notification of authorities or family by smart-phone

In the future, our bodies and smartphones will have innu-merable sensors to monitor our every activity.

Today, we are watched by motion sensors, surveillance cameras, and even x-ray scanners to look into vehicles and buildings. George Orwell might have gotten the year wrong in his landmark book *1984* but the privacy concerns remain and will get potentially even more intrusive than he imagined. Big Brother is watching our every move.

18.1.5   The Star Trek tricorder

Set in the 23rd century, the 1966 TV series *Star Trek* was amaz-ingly prophetic of scientific and medical advances from even

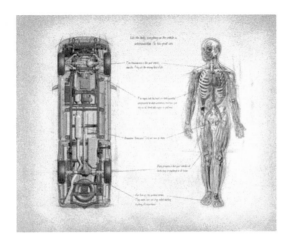

Figure 18.8: Proposed OnStar® health management system.

our 21st century. Here are just a few of the predictions from that series that have already come true:

- Communicator, really just a flip cell phone

- Transparent aluminum, used for that tank holding the whales, now a reality

- Needle-less injection, high pressure air injection, available now for flu shots

- Phasers that stun, essentially a Taser that fires barbs and the electricity causes temporary paralysis

- Universal translators, have you tried Google Translate?

- VISOR, which allows the blind (Geordi) to see, in development today, as are bionic eyes

- Beaming up or teletransportation, analogous to 3D printing, though not for people (yet)

- The tricorder, short for tri-function recorder is also essentially here today

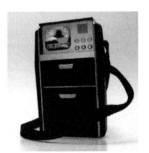

The tricorder is the wireless non-invasive device that *Star Trek's* Dr. Jim "Bones" McCoy used to measure a patient's health. Essentially, the tricorder had some features we take for granted today, including sensors for vital signs, such as

Figure 18.9: Facsimile tricorder, the device used by Dr. James "Bones" McCoy on the TV show *Star Trek* (Modified from JD Hancock/Wikimedia).

heart rate, blood pressure, temperature, oxygen levels, blood glucose, and others, many presently available on your smartphone. Handheld ultrasound devices, like the GE Vscan™ cost less than $10,000 and physicians use them to image everything from the heart and superficial blood vessels, even to include deep tissues. Handheld ultrasound is routinely performed in emergency situations in hospitals today.

In 2012, the X Prize Foundation and San Diego's Qualcomm announced a $10 million prize for developing a tricorder-like health diagnostic device. To win the prize, they require that your tricorder must outperform physicians, weigh no more than 5 pounds, and be able to diagnose 16 medical conditions non-invasively. Ten finalists were announced in 2014, but Qualcomm has been a little slow in announcing a winner, perhaps because they don't want to part with the $10 million.

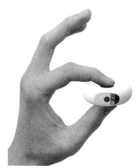

Figure 18.10: A Scanadu Scout™ that obtains non-invasive vital signs within 10 seconds and displays the findings on a smartphone (With permission, Scanadu).

One leading contender is Scanadu, which already has one device, available for $199, that obtains numerous vital signs in just 10 seconds after touching your temple.

A second Scanadu device performs a home urine analysis, diagnosing everything from diabetes to kidney failure to infection. Teleportation, "Beam me up Scotty," and Warp Drive can't be far behind.

Eric Topol, nationally recognized Scripps physician (and medical school classmate of mine), can often be seen demonstrating new wireless health technologies on TV and at conferences. His new book, *The Patient Will See You Now*, is focused just on this subject, what he calls "unplugged digitization, with the smartphone as the hub." I saw Eric there that first day of med school where we were encouraged to use big words. I just call my phone a tricorder.

18.2   Wrap

These are my predictions. I cheated a little because many of these futuristic products are available now. I do have one reliable prediction that I got in a recent fortune cookie, "There will be gigantic unforeseen advances in the near future."

Buckle up.

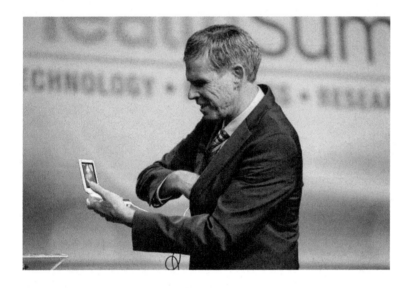

Figure 18.11: Dr. Eric
Topol, of Scripps Health,
demonstrating the GE
Vscan™ ultrasound unit
showing his own heart's
image.

19
Summary

For those who are still watching *Grey's Anatomy* reruns while reading, let me summarize what we have learned, one pearl from each chapter:

1. Live better electrically.

2. We have about 2.5 billion heart beats in our lives, so expect an occasional hiccup.[1]

3. Fainting, which doctors call syncope, is often a warning of a life-threatening arrhythmia. See a doctor.

4. Arrhythmias are simple to treat, just follow the algorithm, and don't listen to computers that are smarter than you.

5. The 24-hour Holter monitor is obsolete and has been replaced with newer and better technology such as the ZIO® Patch and AliveCor Kardia™.

6. CPR is easy, just remember, "Ah, ah, ah, ah, stayin' alive ..."

7. Sudden death and ventricular fibrillation (VF) can be treated with an implantable cardioverter defibrillator (ICD).

8. Your ejection fraction (EF) is more important to know than your cholesterol.

9. Dr. Oz does not work at Scripps and shouldn't be trusted.

10. If it wasn't for a dead cow, warfarin would never have been discovered.

11. Don't stop your blood thinner unless you have a really good reason.

12. Pacemakers without leads are here today.

[1] Electricians are also much better looking than plumbers.

13. The ICD was developed because a friend died suddenly; the three M's—Morowski, Mower and Moss—recognized there ought to be a better way.

14. Ablation has come a long way from open heart surgery and small explosions to today's relatively safe mapping and treatment procedure using catheters.

15. Your best chance of a good result is to pick a hospital and physician with high volume.

16. If you have been diagnosed with atrial fibrillation (AF), get it treated early and often because AF leads to more AF.

17. Heart failure (HF) is worse than cancer, but incredible advances are available today.

18. Everything predicted on *Star Trek* has (or will) come true.

19. Some cardiologists should give up on telling funny jokes.

19.1   *About the author, Steven Higgins, MD, FHRS*

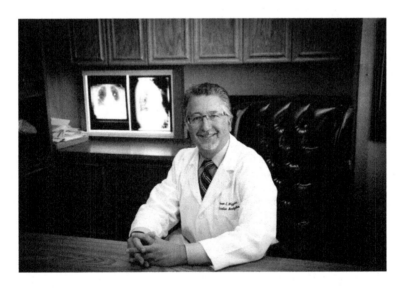

I've been in the cardiac rhythm management field nearly from its inception, about the time that the term cardiac electrophysiologist was invented in the middle of the last century. I've practiced (How do you get to Carnegie Hall? Practice, practice,

practice) clinical cardiac electrophysiology (EP) for more than
30 years at Scripps Memorial Hospital in San Diego.

During that time, Scripps has grown from being a local hospital mostly treating well-heeled residents of beautiful La Jolla,
California, to one of the largest heart-focused hospitals in the
country. Our cardiac program has been ranked in the top 20 for
the past 3 years by *US News & World Report*. Although it seems
that every hospital today has a banner claiming "Best" from
some survey, *U.S. News* is considered the most reliable ranking
of U.S. hospitals, similar to its leadership in college rankings.
Its rankings are devised by a complex formula, part reputation,
part volume, part sophisticated capabilities, and part quality
of care. Being ranked top 20 is a big deal, especially for a hospital that doesn't have a medical school or university to add
to its reputation. Remember that this is 20 out of about 5,000.
Now granted, the Cleveland Clinic, Mayo Clinic, and Harvard
hospitals are ranked ahead of us. I am proud that I have been
the director of Cardiac Electrophysiology at Scripps La Jolla
for more than 30 years and the chairman of the Department
of Cardiology for the past 5 with more than 100 outstanding
cardiologists in our department.

I have published more than 150 peer-reviewed articles or
abstracts in my field, several in the prestigious *New England
Journal of Medicine*. I have also received numerous awards in
the field of EP including the Expert in the Field of Cardiac
Electrophysiology award and the Pioneer in the History of the
Implantable Defibrillator award.

My true enjoyment is taking care of people with heart
rhythm ailments, and I consider saving a life or two my greatest
accomplishment. Along the way, I also like to tell a few jokes
and hope you both learned something and enjoyed *Live Better
Electrically*.

19.2   Acknowledgments

I'd like to thank my friends and colleagues who helped design,
edit, and construct *Live Better Electrically* through their careful
criticism:

- Joe Smith, MD, a genius that I am proud to call a friend

- Claire Kuypers, an EP nurse who has worked with me from the days when we did studies in a little closet in radiology

- Kathy Drennan, NP, my EP nurse practitioner who "volunteered" to read the book cover to cover

- Jim Sparks, a dear friend and colleague who works as a device representative extraordinaire; Jim and I have worked together since 1986

- David Benz (content editing and layout design), Tone Branson (cover design), and Mollie Brumm (copy editing) for their help with designing and editing the book

Finally, I want to thank my wife, Sue. She put up with me working late nights, even sliding food under the closed door like I was in prison. Then, she spent countless hours proofing the various drafts. Sue, as I said at the beginning, thanks for not jumping out on Vail Pass. You have made my life so very special; you are my living valentine.

Steven L. Higgins, MD, FHRS
May 2016

20
Additional resources

The world has changed. Inquisitive readers are more commonly using a search engine for up-to-date information on topics of interest. Thus, a traditional bibliography has little value. Instead, I have listed a limited number of resources culled from books, journals, websites, and guidelines.

Chapter 5: How to document your rhythm problem

- *All the current monitors in more detail*: Higgins, Steven L. "A novel patch for heart rhythm monitoring. Is the Holter monitor obsolete?" *Future Cardiology*, 9(3):325-333, February 2013.

- AliveCor Kardia™: www.alivecor.com.

- ZIO® Patch: www.irhythmtech.com, requires a prescription.

Chapter 7: Arrhythmias 101: Slow and fast

- *EKG interpretation*: Dubin, Dale. *Rapid Interpretation of EKGs*. Tampa, FL: Cover Publishing Company, 2000.

- *Basics on arrhythmias*: http://www.cardiacarrhythmiaassoc.com/#!arrhythmias/c1pna.

- *Ventricular tachycardia*: https://www.scripps.org/services/heart-care__cardiac-arrhythmia-treatment/ventricular-tachycardia.

Chapter 8: Risk factors

- *CAD risk assessment tool*: http://www.cvriskcalculator.com/.

- *AHA heart attack risk calculator*: http://professional.heart.org/professional/GuidelinesStatements/PreventionGuidelines/UCM_457698_Prevention-Guidelines.jsp.

- *Arrhythmia risk factors*: http://www.hrsonline.org/Patient-Resources/Risk-Factors-Prevention.

- *How to calculate your heart's age*: http://www.cnn.com/2015/09/01/health/heart-age-calculator.

Chapter 9: Diet and over-the-counter drugs

- *Omega-3 fatty acid supplements*: Rizos, Evangelos C. "Association Between Omega-3 Fatty Acid Supplementation and Risk of Major Cardiovascular Disease Events." *Journal of the American Medical Association*, 308:1024-1033, 2012. http://jama.jamanetwork.com/article.aspx?articleid=1357266.

- *Dietary supplements*: Cohen, Pieter A. *New England Journal of Medicine*, 366:389-391, 2012. http://www.nejm.org/doi/full/10.1056/NEJMp1113325.

- *Dr. Oz, humorous but detailed review by John Oliver*: https://www.youtube.com/watch?v=TucUMpWWe8A.

Chapter 10: Finding the right doctor

- *Finding the right doctor*: http://www.heart.org/HEARTORG/Conditions/More/MyHeartandStrokeNews/Finding-the-Right-Doctor_UCM_441872_Article.jsp#.Vmev6rgrJhE.

- *Picking a health insurance plan*: http://www.consumerreports.org/cro/2012/09/understanding-health-insurance/index.htm

- *Choosing a heart hospital*: U.S. News & World Report. http://health.usnews.com/best-hospitals/rankings/cardiology-and-heart-surgery.

Chapter 11: Blood thinners and prescription medications

- *NOACs vs. warfarin*: AF meta-analysis in thelancet.com.
  http://williams.medicine.wisc.edu/NOAC_afib_meta_analysis_
  2014.pdf.

- *CHADSVasc score calculator*: www.mdcalc.com.
  http://www.mdcalc.com/cha2ds2-vasc-score-for-atrial-
  fibrillation-stroke-risk/.

- *Comparison of antiarrhythmic drugs*: Tufts University manuscript.
  http://ocw.tufts.edu/data/50/636944.pdf.

- "The problems with Digoxin," CBS News. http://www.cbs
  news.com/news/study-links-heart-medication-digoxin-to-
  deaths/.

Chapter 12: Devices 1: So you need a pacemaker

- *Pacemakers*: Barold, S. Serge et al. *Cardiac Pacemakers and
  Resynchronization Step-by-Step.* Wiley-Blackwell, 2010.

- *Cardiac Resynchronization Therapy (CRT)*: Moss, Arthur J. et al
  (including Higgins, Steven L.). "MADIT-CRT Trial Investigators. Cardiac-resynchronization therapy for the prevention
  of heart-failure events." *New England Journal of Medicine*,
  361:1329-1338, 2009.

- *Leadlessp pacing*: Higgins, Steven L. and Rogers J.D. "Advances in pacing therapy. Examining the potential impact
  of leadless pacing therapy. *Innovations in Cardiac Rhythm
  Management*, 5:1825-1833, 2014.

Chapter 13: So you need a defibrillator

General

- Hayes, D.L. and Zipes D.P. "Cardiac pacemakers and car-
  dioverter defibrillators." In: Libby, P., Bonow R.O., Mann
  D.L., Zipes D.P., eds. *Braunwald's Heart Disease: A Textbook of
  Cardiovascular Medicine*. 8th ed. Chapter 34. Philadelphia, Pa:
  Saunders Elsevier, 2007.

- Higgins, Steven L. *The Implantable Cardioverter Defibrillator. A Videotape and Manual*. Armonk, NY: Futura Publishing Co. Inc, 1997.

- *MADIT study*: Moss, Arthur J. et al. (including Higgins, Steven L.) "Prophylactic implantation of a defibrillator in patients with myocardial infarction and reduced ejection fraction." *New England Journal of Medicine*, 346:877-883, 2002.

- *MADIT II study*: *NBC News* (Higgins). https://www.youtube.com/watch?v=agZCK5Bfz98.

Experts aren't always right

- Lown, Bernard and Axelrod, Paul. "Implanted standby defibrillation." *Circulation*, 46:637, 1972.

History of the ICD

- Cannom, David and Prystowsky, Eric. "The evolution of the Implantable Cardioverter Defibrillator." *PACE*, 27:419-431, 2004. http://www.pacericd.com/documents/ARTICLES/Evolution%20of%20the%20ICD%20PACE%202004.pdf.

- *Indications for an ICD*: Expert Consensus Statement on "Appropriate Use Criteria for Implantable Cardioverter-Defibrillators and Cardiac Resynchronization Therapy." http://www.hrsonline.org/content/download/12357/562699/file/2013_AUC_on-ICD-and-CRT.pdf.

Chapter 14: Ablation

- *Basics of catheter ablation*: http://www.cardiacarrhythmiaassoc.com/#!catheter-ablation/cj7j. http://circ.ahajournals.org/content/106/25/e203.full.

- *Atrial flutter ablation*: http://www.drjohnm.org/2013/08/atrial-flutter-15-facts-you-may-want-to-know/.

- *VT/PVC ablation:* Aliot, E.M. et al. "EHRA/HRS expert consensus on catheter ablation of ventricular arrhythmias." Heart Rhythm, 6:886-933, 2009.

- *Mechanism and ablation*: A great 4-minute video from the Cleveland Clinic. I love the cartoon image of the left heart, PVI, and how it works with that ablation doctor who looks like he is still in high school. `https://www.youtube.com/watch?v=SZ_uIfj-hIQ`.

Chapter 15: Safety and ablation

- *Anesthesia*: `http://emedicine.medscape.com/article/1271543-overview`.

- *Complications*: `http://circ.ahajournals.org/content/128/19/2104.abstract`.

- *Radiation reduction*: Higgins, Steven L. "Integration of fluoroscopy images in a 3-D mapping system reduces fluoroscopy exposure during catheter ablation procedures." *Diagnostic Interventional Cardiology*, 5:25, 2013.

- *Left atrial appendage occlusion*: "The Lariat™ Needs Lassoing." `http://www.medscape.com/viewarticle/844184`.

Chapter 16: Atrial fibrillation

- *AF resources including 3D mapping*: `https://www.biosensewebster.com/community-outreach/afib.aspx`.

- *A simple book on AF for novices*: Stone, C. and Trimborn, E. *Atrial Fibrillation: What You Need to Know*. Available in electronic format only.

Chapter 17: Heart failure

- *Basics*: Jaski, B. *The 4 Stages of Heart Failure*. Minneapolis, MN: Cardiotest Publishing, 2015.

- *Advanced*: Yancy, W. et al. 2013 ACCF/AHA Guidelines for the Management of Heart Failure. *Circulation*, 128:e240-e327, 2013.

Chapter 18: Future advances—some available today

- *Overview of gene and cell therapy*: `http://www.asgct.org/`

general-public/educational-resources/gene-therapy-and-cell-
therapy-defined.

- *Star Trek predicted the future*: http://entertainment.howstuff
works.com/10-star-trek-technologies.htm.

- *The future of medicine*: Topol, Eric. *The Patient Will See You
Now*. New York, NY: Basic Books. Perseus, 2015.

21

Index